THE AMEN SOLUTION

GET HEALTHY

with **THE BRAIN DOCTOR'S** *Wife*

Coaching Guide

TANA AMEN, B.S.N.

Published by MindWorks Press, Newport Beach, California.

A Division of Amen Clinics, Inc.

www.amenclinics.com

Author: Tana Amen, BSN

Layout and Design: Jaclyn Frattali

Cover Art: Rick Cortez

Printed in China

OTHER BOOKS BY TANA AMEN

EAT HEALTHY WITH THE BRAIN DOCTOR'S WIFE COOKBOOK, MindWorks Press, 2011

CHANGE YOUR BRAIN, CHANGE YOUR BODY COOKBOOK, MindWorks Press, 2010

Dedication:

To Tamara and Jenny.

Your stories are why I do what I do!

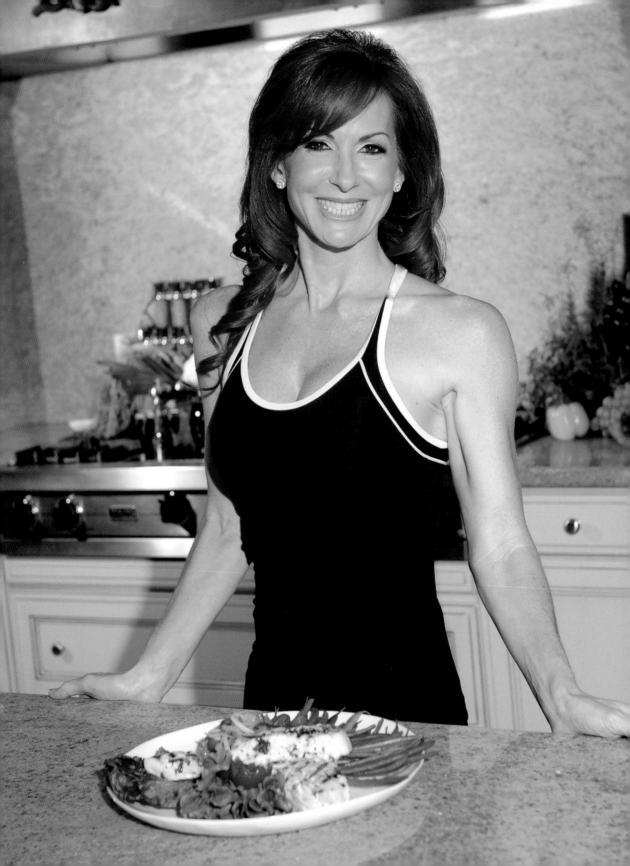

Table of Contents

I am 32 years old. I have been suffering with an unexplained autoimmune disorder for years. When I was 25, my doctor thought I had Lupus. When that was ruled out, they tested me for Rheumatoid Arthritis and then several other diseases. Eventually, I fell into the catch-all diagnosis of "Fibromyalgia." But I don't know many people with Fibromyalgia who spend three hours every day in the bathroom, exhausted and in pain.

Two years ago my diarrhea escalated from one to two times a day to an exhausting five or six times a day. It was painful and left me feeling like I always was running on empty. It was affecting my relationship with my children, my ability to be employed and the intimacy with my husband. I began to live my life around my diarrhea, often waking several hours earlier than normal just to have time to "deal with it." Most days I took two showers just to feel clean. This became a debilitating way to live.

This was not the only pain I lived with. My joints were swollen. My knuckles would split and bleed when I changed my baby's diaper. I had shooting pain in my back from walking up my stairs. My daily naps grew increasingly longer. I was unable to tolerate working or being on my feet for very long. This affected my opportunities for employment. I felt guilty that I never took my kids to the park to play on sunny days.

Yet another visit to the doctor had me going through another battery of tests to rule out Rheumatoid Arthritis (again), Celiac-Sprue, Crohn's Disease, and Irritable Bowel Syndrome. During my initial visit, it was discovered that my triglycerides were 295 (normal is less than 150), my cholesterol was 258 (less than 200 is optimal), and my blood pressure was 139/96 (below 120/80 is optimal)! My weight had crept up to 206 pounds after having my second child, and I am only 5 feet 4 inches tall. My vitamin D level was less than 20 (optimal is 50-90). The doctor said nothing about a lifestyle change.

Instead, I walked out of the doctor's office with a prescription for a statin to help lower my cholesterol. But, I didn't want to start taking another medication at age 32. Instinctively, I knew that if I just gave in and started taking a handful of pills without changing my lifestyle I would become more and more unhealthy. I have two small children. I HAD to be healthy for my children, but I had NO IDEA where to start.

It was then that I called Tana. I knew that I could call her for sound advice about nutrition. I had been hearing about the Amen principles, but I had been resistant to change until this point. The first thing Tana suggested was that I continue to follow through with my medical testing . . . AND that I make radical changes in my lifestyle. She suspected that I had a food allergy so she recommended that I try an "elimination diet" while I was waiting for the results of my tests.

I followed Tana's advice, and I figured that it would take several weeks before I saw any kind of difference. But after just TWO days of following the principles from the "The Amen Solution," I awoke to a normal bowel movement! I didn't spend hours in the bathroom! My daughter said, "Mommy, you don't stink." How could years of suffering appear to be reversed after only a few days of nutritional eating and taking a few supplements? And it isn't only my bowels that have benefitted! I lost 22 pounds in six weeks, and the swelling and pain in my joints is virtually gone. I'm now living with less pain, more rest, and a higher quality of life—and this happened almost overnight!

It breaks my heart now when I see people needlessly suffering. I sit in the doctor's office and see so many overweight people, all in pain. It's often the same people each time I go. I told my doctor about the program I am on. She said, "It isn't possible. You still need medication. Nutrition and lifestyle will never be enough." I became so angry! It was then that I realized how overweight she was herself. I said, "Really, then how do you think I have lost so much weight and feel so much less pain with this program in such a short time? I feel great!" I wondered how much weight she had lost recently.

I'd love to say it's magic, but it's really logic. After Tana clearly explained the principles of nutrition and food allergies and sensitivities, I realized that I had been poisoning my body. Once I stopped the poisoning and started getting real nutrition, my body responded immediately! I cannot put into words the relief I've been blessed with.

Gratefully Yours,

Tamara G.

Reno, NV

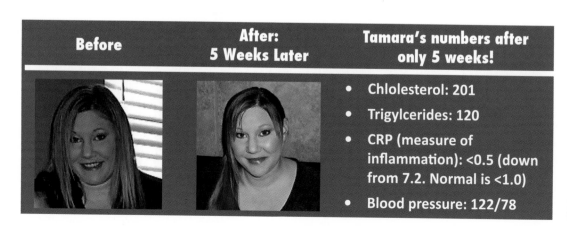

Before	After: 5 Weeks Later	Tamara's numbers after only 5 weeks!
		• Chlolesterol: 201
		• Trigylcerides: 120
		• CRP (measure of inflammation): <0.5 (down from 7.2. Normal is <1.0)
		• Blood pressure: 122/78

INTRODUCTION

If you are purchasing this book, you likely realize that it is a companion to *The Amen Solution*, which was written by my husband, Dr. Daniel Amen, a neuroscientist, psychiatrist, and brain-imaging specialist. However, you may not realize that studying and teaching nutrition and fitness have been a passion of mine for years. In fact, I often receive calls from friends and neighbors asking me for advice about health and nutrition. Also, when I am at lectures with my husband, people sometimes approach me to ask questions about nutrition and supplements. I hear them say things like, "Ask the brain doctor's wife, she prob-

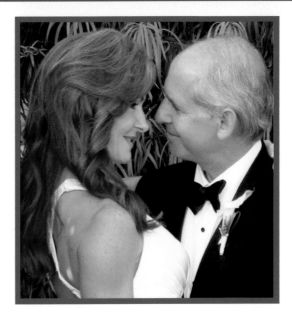

ably knows." Frankly, my husband thinks I am a nerd because of how much I love science and physiology, so this name came to stick. Now I am known as "The Brain Doctor's Wife."

But more important, I am a person who has lived a life that was both deeply affected by making many of the nutritional and fitness mistakes that harm so many people and a life that has been entirely transformed by following the principles that are outlined in this book. So, it is with my whole heart and all of my own experience that I promise that this guide will transform your life. I am confident that after the first 30 days you will be so hooked on the changes in your mental clarity, energy, vitality—and even the size of your butt!—that you will not want to give up following the recommendations in this book. Better yet, follow these recommendations for at least 12 weeks and they will become so ingrained in your psyche that they will become a part of your identity! Once that happens, there is no turning back and there will be no stopping you!

PREDATING THE "BRAIN DOCTOR'S WIFE"

"A wise man learns from his mistakes, but a wiser man learns from someone else's."
- Unknown

My husband and I live an amazing, passion-filled life, and health and nutrition are at the core. But my story has not always been centered on health, fitness, and vitality! On the contrary, I grew up in a garden variety dysfunctional American family. My mother was a single, working parent who usually worked several jobs to make ends meet. She often struggled with her own weight and health issues when I was young. Meals were a combination of survival (I just had to figure out what was available to eat and make it happen) and using food to comfort myself. I was an anxious kid who was left alone a lot and learned to survive.

Since we were poor and my mother knew very little about nutrition at that time, breakfast was usually Cap'n Crunch or Pop-Tarts. Lunch was whatever pseudo-food was being served at school. My afternoon snack often was Nestle's Quik chocolate milk and another bowl of cereal. Dinner might be warm tortillas with butter and sugar or, if there was someone around to help me turn on the oven, a frozen pot pie (this tells you how old I am since we didn't even have a microwave!).

Given this history and my genetics, I should have been fat and sick at an early age . . . and this nearly became a self-fulfilling prophecy. Both of my grandmothers had Type II Diabetes. There was cancer, heart disease, and dementia on both sides of my family. Fortunately, though, every cloud has a silver lining. I was never overweight. As a matter of fact, I was a very skinny kid. By the time I was 14 years old I became so disgusted with the chronic obesity and health issues plaguing my family that it terrorized me into action. I loved my family, but I didn't want to be anything like them when it came to health and fitness.

At the time, though, I did not know how to truly break the cycle that hurt my family. I just figured that exercising would send me down a different path. An avid exerciser right out of high school, I began working out obsessively in the gym. However, I still knew little about diet and nutrition. Since I worked out so hard, I believed that I could eat whatever I wanted and still remain lean as long as I managed the quantity of those foods. I never took the quality of those food choices into consideration.

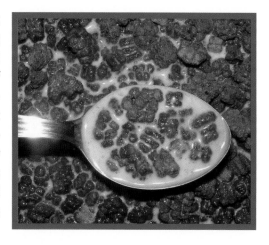

But, it didn't take long for the effects of that lifestyle to wreak havoc on my health. Eating a lot of processed foods, simple carbs, and caffeine can't be countered by two and half hours in the gym. Actually, the excessive exercise was collaborating with my lousy diet to make me sick! Though I was thin and appeared fit on the outside, I was tearing my body apart on the inside. By the time I was 23 years old, I was diagnosed with thyroid cancer that had metastasized into my lymph nodes. After a couple of surgeries, several radiation treatments, and six years of frustration with thyroid imbalances, I finally felt that I had that problem licked and that I was on my way to beginning the rest of my life!

I made the decision (so I thought) to eat healthier by eating according to the food pyramid. But a few years later I found out that I had to have my gall bladder removed! Then I discovered that I was insulin resistant, had high triglycerides, and had high cholesterol! At that time I was only 118 pounds and had just 13 percent body fat, so my doctor said it must be genetic.

Unsatisfied and unwilling to go on more medication, I went on a quest for the answer! Through research, I discovered that most of what I had learned about nutrition from school was a joke—and a bad one! I came to understand that our food-pyramid-centered sense of nutrition is driven by the food industry and by the mega agribusiness world. It became clear to me that I was throwing fuel on the fire of my unraveling health with the foods I was eating.

My quest also brought me to the world of health care. I worked as a neurosurgical ICU nurse for many years where I saw the effects of poor lifestyle choices, with food topping the charts, on a daily basis. I also have long been a health advocate. These careers began for me when I attended college at Loma Linda University and worked at their Medical Center. This institution is known for its emphasis on treating the "whole person" and for the longevity statistics of the community it serves—despite the fact that it is located in intensely smoggy San Bernardino, California.

Not coincidentally, Loma Linda is a Seventh Day Adventist institution. The Seventh Day Adventists adhere to a strict vegetarian diet of whole foods, a life of temperance, and a belief that you can't treat an individual part of a person but that you need to treat the person from a bio-psycho-social-spiritual perspective. As a result, nutrition was an important part of my training at Loma Linda.

In addition to being a nurse and a health advocate, my personal struggle and ultimate victory over years of chronic health issues, battles with cravings, and struggles for energy and vitality that are not fueled by caffeine and sugar have given me a voracious appetite for continuing my education in the field of nutrition and fitness. Unfortunately for me, I have tried a lot of crazy tactics in this pursuit. Fortunately for you, I have learned a lot through this process of trial and error and research.

Now, with this book, my ultimate success means that you do not have to reinvent the wheel! Instead, it is my privilege to have created this book so that I can help you on this initial leg of your journey to a better brain, a smaller waist, and many years of living thinner, smarter, and happier.

To this end, I have designed this book so that it is full of useful tables that are full of practical information. For those of you who don't have the time or the inclination to want to know the "why" behind the principles in this book, you can read these sections first and just learn the "how." But, for those of you who want to dig a little deeper and learn the "why" as well, I have incorporated a special feature into this book called "NERD NOTES!" Here, you will find a deeper, but still palatable, explanation about the "why."

Above all, I want to share with you how it is possible that I am now in my forties and I am experiencing the highest level of energy, passion, and joy that I have ever experienced! I truly live my day-to-day life according to the principles contained in this book.

It is my great hope that this book will show you that The Amen Solution is about eating in a way that provides you access to a fountain of youth similar to the one that I have found. It's about helping you recover and heal by stopping the poisoning and taking a giant leap into an amazing world of health and vitality! Just remember that if I can achieve this level of fitness, health, and vitality in spite of having my thyroid and gall bladder removed, overcoming cancer, and being insulin resistant, there is no reason you can't do it also.

So, right now, I challenge you to set aside all of the excuses and limiting beliefs that have been holding you back and to take a leap of faith by dedicating the next 12 weeks to achieving outstanding results! Oh, by the way . . . check out my mother at age 64. She also feels and looks better than she has in decades! She is a shining example that The Amen Solution works!

Mom Before - Age 50

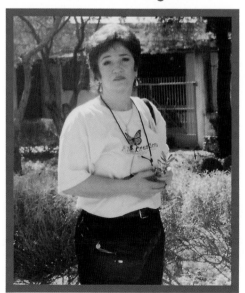

Mom After - Age 64

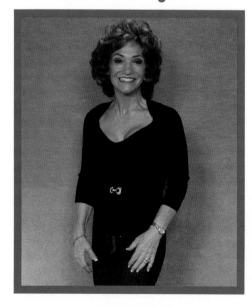

Tana's Typical Day of Nutrition

My total calories remain between 1650 – 1850, depending upon my activity level and how hard I've worked out.

16 ounces of water upon waking

Breakfast: (Within one hour of waking up)

"Brain Balancing Smoothie" made with 1/2 cup of organic berries or cherries, 1/8 avocado, a handful of spinach (Work with me here! I promise you won't taste it!), a scoop of dried greens, 4 - 8 ounces of coconut water or unsweetened almond milk, 15 - 20 grams of protein powder and a few drops of Stevia. I also add a few "super foods" such as bee pollen, aloe vera gel, raw cocoa, etc. I usually follow this with a cup of green or herbal tea.

Approximately 220 - 250 calories

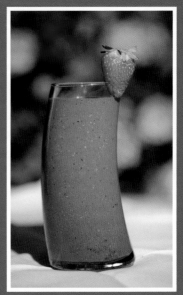

Mid-Morning Snack: 1/4 cup raw nuts or seeds
Approximately 150 calories

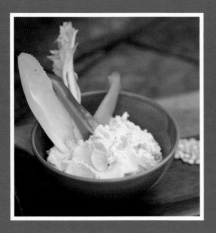

Meal #2: (About 3 hours after breakfast)

By this time I usually have consumed another 16 ounces of water with fresh squeezed lemon juice.

2 - 3 cups of raw, chopped veggies with 2 Tbsp hummus, baba ghanouj or salsa; 2 - 3 ounces of lean protein (usually tuna, salmon or shrimp); 1 Tbsp of chopped, raw almonds or walnuts.

Approximately 340 – 400 calories

Mid-Afternoon Snack: 1/4 cup raw nuts or seeds; raw veggies or 1/2 apple
Approximately 150 - 180 calories

Meal #3:

By this time I have consumed at least another 16 ounces of water.

Option #1 - Arugula Salad with Raspberries. Top with either 1/8 avocado or 2 tsp of raw seeds (chia, flax, hemp, or pumpkin seeds are a great addition to a salad).

Approximately 220 – 350 calories

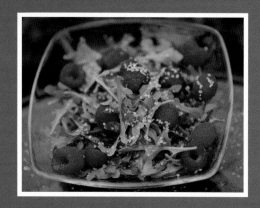

Option #2 - If I am on the run, I have another "Brain Balancing Smoothie" with 1/2 apple, 1/2 grapefruit or pear, 1/2 carrot, 1/2 cucumber, one scoop of dried greens, 10 - 15 grams of protein powder, and 1 Tbsp flax or pumpkin seeds.

Approximately 250 calories

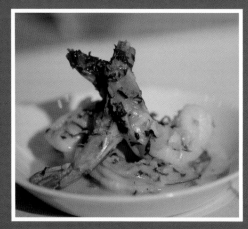

Dinner:

By this time I have consumed at least another 16 ounces of water.

1 1/2 cups of shredded spaghetti squash or Shiritaki noodle "pasta" with tomato basil sauce containing 2 - 3 ounces of lean protein (shrimp or ground turkey); a large green salad with 1 Tbsp of olive oil dressing; 1 - 2 cups of steamed broccoli; 1 cup of caffeine-free herbal tea with Stevia sweetener.

Approximately 280 – 350 calories

Dessert:

By this time I have consumed at least another 16 ounces of water.

Option #1 - 1/4 cup "Avocado Gelato" (It's to die for, I promise!)

Approximately 125 calories

Option #2 - 1/2 of a "Brain on Joy" coconut bar (Can be found on www.amenclinics.com.)

Approximately 70 calories

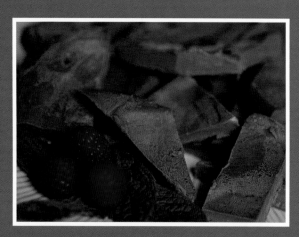

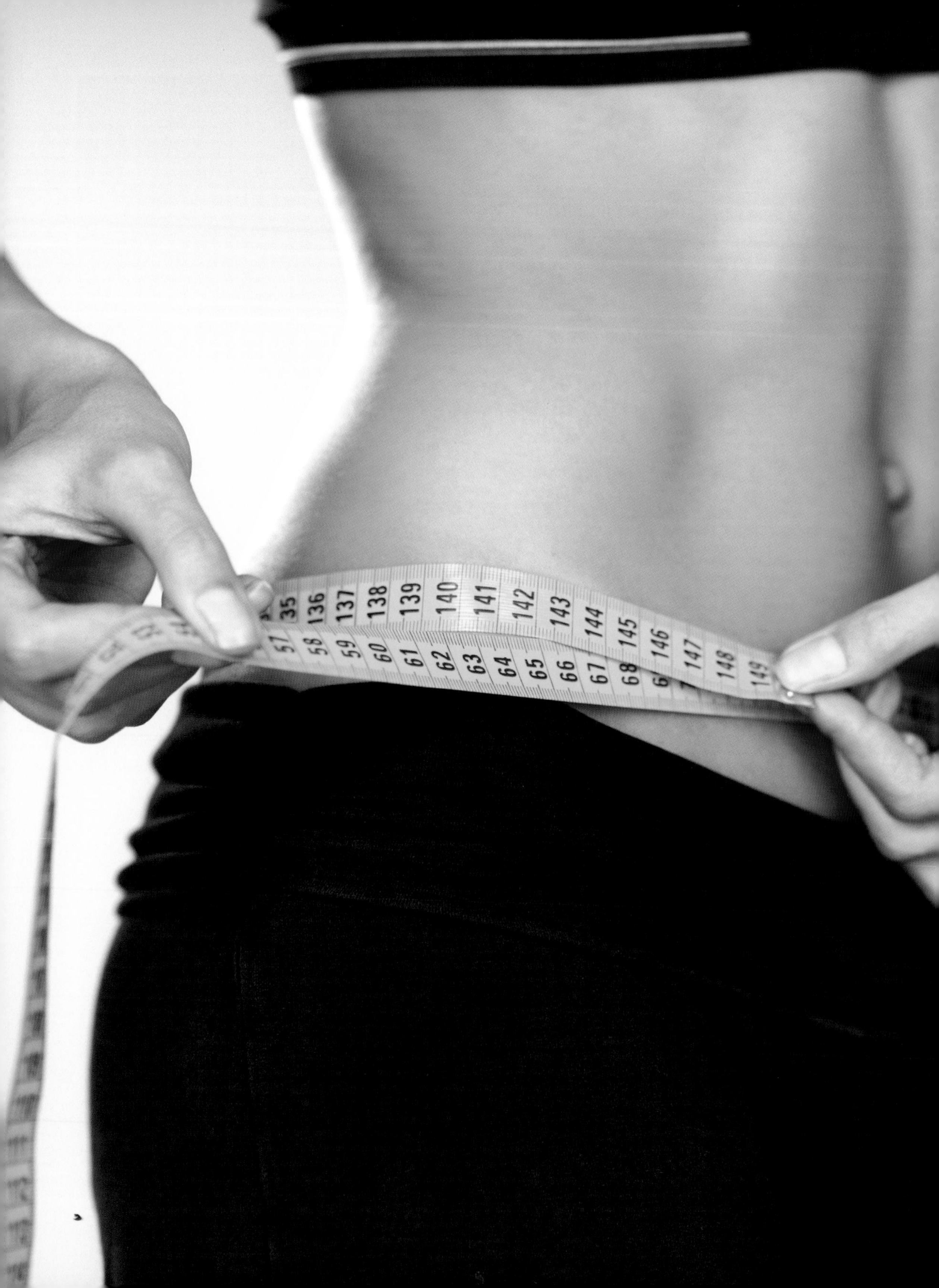

Chapter 1

WHY "D-I-E"TS FAIL
and *The Amen Solution* Works

WHY "D-I-E"TS FAIL and *The Amen Solution* Works

I absolutely hate to diet! The first three letters in the word diet are D-I-E! I don't like feeling deprived, grumpy, or tired, and I bet you don't either. Most diets are designed to give you instant gratification in the form of immediate weight loss. When you go on a diet and radically cut your calories and aggressively begin restricting foods, you temporarily get results. But these diets don't take the "big" picture into account. They are just a quick way to sell books or supplements and make you happy by shedding a lot of weight quickly (which is not healthy). Unfortunately, this way of dieting never takes care of your body's underlying issues with insulin resistance and sugar addiction, and it never educates you about a permanent lifestyle change.

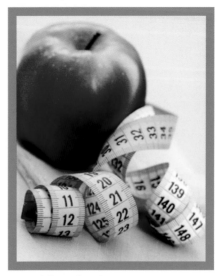

Another problem with most diets is that they don't change as you change. As you become leaner and begin to shed pounds, you must continually adjust your program. A 200-pound person can't eat the same number of calories as a 250-pound person and expect to continue to lose weight—or to even maintain the weight loss achieved—unless that person increases their metabolism through increased activity. You must recalculate the number of calories you need to continue on your journey. If you are hitting plateaus, you must stop and consider that it may be time to adjust your program. What works in the beginning of your program eventually will change and need to be adjusted.

In addition, most diets leave you feeling hungry and deprived. When this happens, you must use sheer willpower to stick to your diet. You will do it for a while, but eventually your internal navigation system will kick in and "redirect the course." We are hardwired to seek satiety, not deprivation. This means that you cannot sustain a diet that makes you feel deprived because your body's natural hormonal response eventually will override even the most determined willpower. It is a simple matter of survival and genetic wiring. You are not designed to diet, and I bet you're glad to hear that!

In fact, humans are biologically hardwired to gain weight! Sounds ominous, I know. But it's not if you understand how we were designed. Never in history have we had such an abundance of food or the ability to store food as we do now. Historically, food was a scarcity, so fat storage was a matter of survival, and storing it made passing on your DNA to your offspring easier. If you were in starvation mode, your genetics determined that you were not fit to procreate. Hence, "survival of the fittest" meant that you had to have a little fat. But this doesn't mean you are destined to be obese. Understanding how your biology works will give you the key to unleash your metabolism and give you boundless energy!

Knowing your biology also helps you to understand why you have such a hard time losing weight . . . and keeping it off. The simple answer is that your metabolism has literally been hijacked! Most of what we were taught in school about the food pyramid is complete garbage and sets you up for failure. It is driven by the agribusiness and mega-food companies.

To see this, we could go back thousands of years and compare the agricultural evolution to increasing disease. In the times prior to farming, our ancestors did not have the widespread food-related problems that plague our society since they had no choice. There was no such thing as processed food, bread, pasta, high fructose corn syrup, cheap oils, and fast food. Foods like these are made from simple, refined carbohydrates and cheap oils that are high in omega-6 fatty acids. (You do need some omega-6 fatty acids in your diet, but it's important to get the proper ratio of omega-6 to omega-3 fatty acids.) These foods not only increase inflammation, they create insulin resistance as well.

But, for our purposes, we will stick to the last 100 years. Since the Industrial Revolution, obesity, diabetes, heart disease, and cancer have skyrocketed. Why? Because we began mass producing food (which often requires the use of harmful hormones, antibiotics, and genetic modification) and packaging it for extended shelf life. This means that we now are eating more than triple the amount of inflammation-causing foods than at any other time in human history.

Interestingly, we haven't actually altered the amount of food we consume all that much, but we have dramatically altered the quality of the food we consume. (Of course this doesn't include those of you who succumb to Super Sizing. You are eating a whole lot more food!) But, for the most part, the same volume of food from the typical American diet of today contains several hundred more calories than the same volume of food from 100 years ago! This is a direct result of processing, sugar, and cheap oils.

This really is brain science!

Fad diets are the antithesis of *The Amen Solution* and will set you up for failure!

- **Most diets make you feel lousy after a couple of days and cause "mental fog." If you feel tired, grumpy, and unfocused, then your brain is not functioning near its capacity. Chances are you are experiencing spikes and drops in blood sugar that result in insulin surges . . . this is NOT a good thing!**

- **If it's bad for your brain and focus, then it's bad for your body too. This means that your body also is not functioning near its potential.**

- **Fad, restrictive diets usually harm your long-term health and metabolism because they cause systemic inflammation and hormonal imbalance. Ultimately, you gain more weight than you lose.**

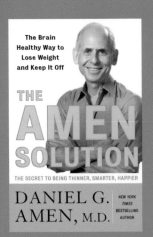

The Brain Healthy Way to Lose Weight and Keep It Off

THE **AMEN SOLUTION**

THE SECRET TO BEING THINNER, SMARTER, HAPPIER

DANIEL G. AMEN, M.D.

NEW YORK TIMES BESTSELLING AUTHOR

The Amen Solution **is different because it emphasizes foods that:**

- **Optimize brain function**

- **Decrease systemic inflammation**

- **Increase satiety**

- **Break food addictions by balancing the hormones of hunger and satiety**

- **Offer high-quality calories**

- **Are consumable in greater quantities because they are micro-nutrient rich yet calorie sparse so you get more "bang for your buck"**

- **Provide a lifestyle of eating that will have you feeling energized and satisfied instead of deprived**

In addition, the following tips and explanations are the reason that we have had such enormous success with *The Amen Solution.*

1. **Never allow yourself to become too hungry when you are actively trying to lose weight.** Be sure to eat between four and six small meals throughout the day.

2. **Break your addiction to sugar and simple carbs immediately!** Otherwise, you will fight the battle of the bulge forever. Do this by eating small amounts of protein and healthy fats with each meal and by increasing the "volume" of your meals by adding LOTS of vegetables and a little fruit to your diet. Do not go all day without eating protein! In fact, increasing your protein throughout the day will automatically rev your metabolism and enhance weight loss. You will be amazed at how quickly you lose your cravings if you follow this formula. But please remember that . . .

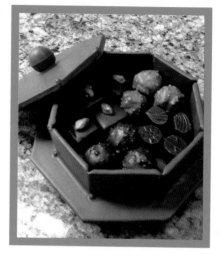

- A healthy, active person may be able to eat a little more protein, but someone with kidney disease or diabetes likely needs a more protein-restricted diet.

- Animal protein is not the only source of protein. Nuts, seeds, vegetarian protein powders and greens also add a significant amount of protein to your diet.

3. **When calories and nutritional information are not available, use the "eyeball method" for estimating your protein intake.** While actively trying to lose weight, you can eat a piece of lean protein about the size and width of your palm with each meal. Once you begin losing weight, or reach your goal weight, you may wish to decrease this amount. I find this to be a lot of protein for my taste. I prefer more veggies and lighter fare . . . unless I am feeling unusually hungry, like after working out.

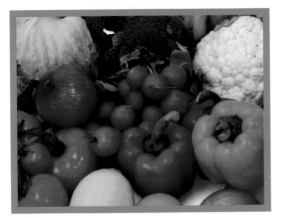

4. **70 percent of your diet should consist of "live," whole, *unprocessed*, water-rich foods.** This primarily means vegetables and fruits. These foods will fill you up quickly with volume, but they are very low in calories. Many vegetables require nearly as much energy for digestion as they contain, and they are packed with phytonutrients.

5. **Eat small amounts of *raw*, unsalted nuts and seeds throughout the day (but not more than 1/2 cup total for the day for your snacks, less for smaller people).** These healthy fats don't make you fat. **SUGAR** makes you fat by spiking insulin and causing insulin resistance. In fact, you need a substantial amount of healthy fats in your diet to prevent "gluconeogenisis" (the conversion of protein to sugar . . . protein in the form of your muscles!) when you start losing weight. The last thing you want is for that weight loss to come at the expense of your hard-earned muscles.

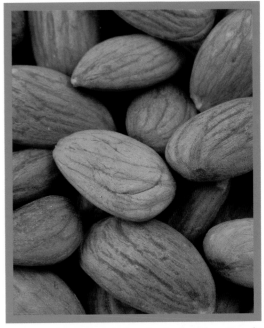

But nuts and seeds are calorie dense, so pay attention to total calorie intake. Don't unconsciously grab a handful and not measure.

6. **Check in with your body regularly to see if it's time to adjust your program.** It may be time to reduce your calorie intake, which means increasing your veggies and fruit and decreasing the fats and proteins a bit. When I first started eating this way, I ate A LOT! I ate five or six small meals each day, and I felt great. But, after a few weeks, I began to feel very full and heavy. I had plateaued. I adjusted by reducing the amount of protein slightly, and I began eating four or five meals each day. I felt amazing again, and my energy went through the roof. Listen to your body!

A Note About Plateaus . . .

When you make any type of dramatic change to your daily eating regimen, your body eventually will adjust and this can lead to those devastating plateaus that undermine the efforts of people who try to lose weight on a typical fad diet. Unlike diets, The Amen Solution takes human biology into account and recognizes that plateaus are often a normal part of the process in a healthy weight-loss program. This means that you should not equate plateaus with failure, but that you should make an honest assessment of where you are in your program. If you have been following The Amen Solution principles and you suddenly hit a plateau, it could mean several things.

A. Initially you may lose weight rapidly as a result of detoxification. When you remove the source of poisoning, your body instantly will respond by decreasing the inflammation. Eventually, it will stabilize and weight loss will take on a slower and steadier pace. Don't be discouraged. This is healthy!

B. Plateaus sometimes occur as a way for the body to adjust to the rapid loss of toxins from the fat cells. Since fat cells store toxic material, your body needs time to clear the waste away. You can override this natural process and "diet" through it, but you will likely put the weight back on, and then some! The Amen Solution is a healthy lifestyle that takes this process into account. Increasing your water intake, consuming more greens or green drinks, and/or participating in activities that cause you to sweat a little more, such as saunas and exercise, will usually help. This process lasts for only one or two weeks.

C. If you have lost a significant amount of weight and you have been eating a lot of animal protein, it may be time to adjust your program and decrease your intake of animal protein a bit, replacing it with more wholesome choices. You will still need to get regular "doses" of protein throughout the day, just in smaller portions. Also, consider eating more veggies and vegetarian sources of protein.

D. It may be time to make an honest assessment of how you have been progressing. Are you journaling? Have you been slipping into old habits? Many times when I speak with people at this critical juncture, I will question them repeatedly about what they are doing differently. They often will say they aren't doing anything differently. But, by about the third time I ask, they suddenly remember the chocolate cake they ate on the weekend . . . and the popcorn at the movies!

E. Having a coach or mentor can help you through these plateaus. At the very least, doing the program with a friend or partner often will keep you more accountable and make it more fun.

7. **Go slow! Losing weight too quickly causes a rapid release of the toxic materials that have been stored in your fat cells.** This burdens the body and can cause significant health issues and systemic inflammation. This in turn drives your body to "do something" about this problem, usually by regaining the weight by increasing your cravings. Losing weight slowly, 1-2 pounds per week, gives the liver and the rest of the body ample time to process these toxins and dispose of them appropriately. Also, losing weight slowly gives you a chance to adjust to the "new you" and to make this change permanent on a psychological level. However, don't panic if you shed pounds quickly in the beginning as long as you are not restricting calories too much and you are drinking a lot of water. You may be detoxifying and eliminating. Everyone is different.

8. **Stay hydrated! Drink half of your body weight in ounces.** If If you are 160 pounds, you should be drinking 80 ounces of water per day. When you increase your protein, you will cause an automatic increase in water loss. You do not want to get dehydrated because dehydration often makes people think they are hungry. Increasing your water intake also will help your body to process and flush out toxins as you lose weight. And drinking water before a meal increases your feeling

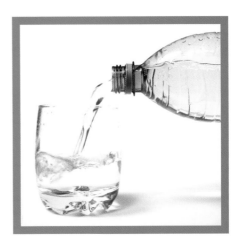

of satiety, causing you to desire less food. So, while we want to see the scale moving down, we don't want it to be water weight. This is meant to be a healthy program, for life!

A Note About Plastic Water Bottles . . .

There are a lot of rumors and misunderstandings circulating about the evils of the dioxins and the phthalates that are found in our plastic bottles and dishes. Since so much of the water that we consume comes out of plastic bottles, we need to touch on this issue for a moment.

Dioxins, which are compounds that are highly toxic to humans, are commonly believed to be created in the process of combustion. However, they are not known to be released in water bottles. Phthalates, which are chemicals known to interrupt endocrine signals and mimic human hormones, are added to some water bottles to give them flexibility. However, this seems to be more of a health hazard when plastics are heated.

The takeaway for me is this:

- *Do* replace plastic water bottles and dishes when possible. (There are environmental reasons for doing this as well.)
- *Don't* get too hung up on this if you aren't always able to do so.

- *Do* drink lots of water even if it means that you occasionally have to buy water in plastic bottles.
- *Don't* store plastic water bottles in your car, wash them in the dishwasher, or heat any plastic dishes in the microwave.

Most Americans are chronically dehydrated and this is a precursor to many diseases in the body. The downsides of dehydration far outweigh the risk of occasionally drinking out of a plastic bottle!

9. **Move your body!** One of the keys to success is to become more active. If you have been doing nothing, start with walking and then increase as you feel capable. If you are more active, try adding circuit training or strength training to your program. Yoga and swimming are great choices as well. Increasing your activity level will enhance your mood and decrease your desire to "mindlessly munch."

[How much protein do you need?]

The average daily protein intake of a healthy individual should be approximately .8 grams of protein per kilogram (.8g/kg) of your body weight. A kilogram is 2.2 pounds.

1. Figure out your weight in kilograms (your weight divided by 2.2)

2. Take your weight in kilograms and multiply it by .8

3. Divide this number equally by the number of meals that you eat throughout the day to determine how much protein you should eat with each meal (this doesn't need to include snacks) . . . and remember that this is an estimate. It's not a big deal if you go a little over or a little under.

For all intents and purposes, we are giving you a way to estimate how much protein to add to your meals through the consumption of meat or supplements. But, remember that meat, protein powders, and protein bars are not the only sources of protein. You will receive a substantial amount of protein from greens, nuts, seeds, and other vegetarian sources.

This does not take into consideration individual health considerations, such as renal disorders, or the increased needs of people with elevated metabolic demands. If you have special health considerations, be sure to consult with your physician.

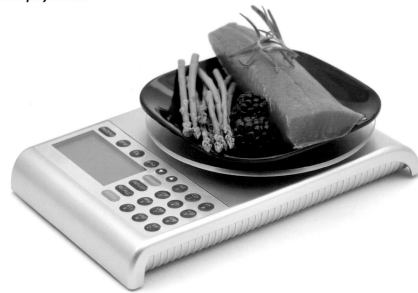

NERD NOTE!
Your Building Blocks

"Macronutrients" describe the proteins, fats, and carbohydrates that make up the nutrition we eat. They all provide some level of fuel, but they are not all equal.

- *Protein* provides the greatest level of satiety and requires the most energy expenditure to digest. It also causes your gut to release the hormone PYY, which improves your sensitivity to the hormone leptin. This sends a message to the brain that you are full. Protein also stimulates the release of glucagon, which is a hormone that has the opposite effect of insulin. Glucagon helps stabilize blood sugar and prevents energy crashes by causing the liver to release stored glucose for energy.

- *Fats* (healthy) also increase satiety by stimulating the release of PYY, but they are second to protein. However, healthy fats are essential for many of the complex functions of the body, including proper brain function, hormone synthesis and cholesterol reduction (That's right! Healthy fats are essential!). Healthy fats also are necessary for preventing oxidative damage and degenerative nerve disorders. In addition, healthy fat is essential in the absorption of many nutrients, vitamins, and minerals. So, it's a good idea to take your supplements with a meal containing a little healthy fat.

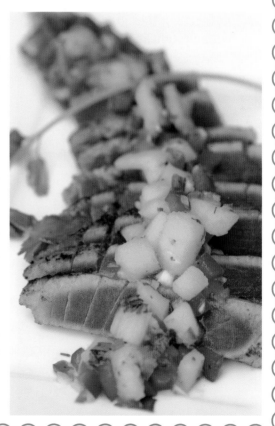

- *Complex carbohydrates* provide energy more quickly than proteins and fats and are quickly used by the brain and body. All carbohydrates, complex or otherwise, must be broken down to their simplest form (glucose or fructose) in order to cross the intestinal lining and make their way into the bloodstream. Vegetables are a form of complex carbohydrates that are very low in sugar and very high in fiber and micronutrients. This makes them an excellent source of energy. Fruit, though, is a touchy subject since it is so high in sugar. Eating fruit in excess or consuming it in a form that removes its fiber, such as juice, can be like injecting a massive bolus of fructose into your body...which is toxic to your liver! But, eaten in moderation and in its whole form, fruit is an excellent source of energy, very satisfying, and filled with fiber, micronutrients, and phytonutrients. It's the fiber packaging that makes fruit "God's guilt-free candy."

- *Some grains and legumes* can be a good source of energy, especially for vegetarians. They are complex carbohydrates that also have a moderate amount of protein. However, most people would do best to avoid gluten as much as possible, and many people have unknown food sensitivities to the proteins in other grains and legumes. (We will talk more about discovering hidden food allergies later.)

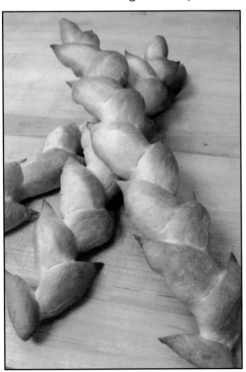

- *Simple carbohydrates* provide instant energy. **This is not a good thing!** Simple or refined carbs such as breads, baked goods, and sugar are poor choices for increasing satiety. They spike insulin levels quickly, cause insulin resistance, increase inflammation, and leave you craving more carbs. They also increase triglycerides and cholesterol and muffle the signal sent from the hunger/satiety hormones ghrelin and leptin, which are responsible for letting you know when you are hungry and when your hunger has been satisfied. The more sugar and simple carbs you eat, the hungrier you will be!

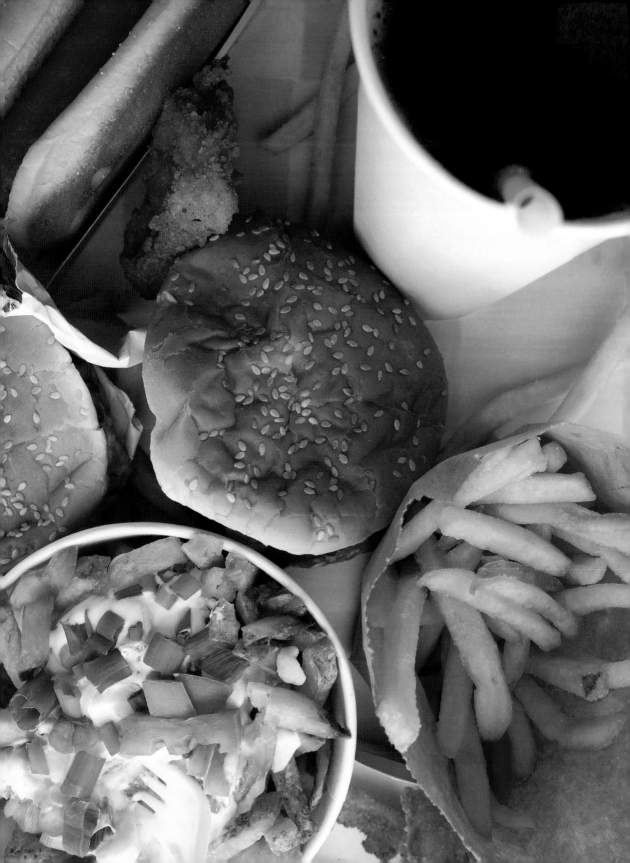

Chapter 2

THE TOXIC TRUTH: Foods That Destroy Your Health

Chapter 2

|||||||||||||||||||||||||||||||||||||||||||||||||||||||||||||||||||||||||||||||||||||||||||||||||||||||||||||||||||||

THE TOXIC TRUTH: Foods That Destroy Your Health

Sweet Death

If you've ever tasted the dessert "Death by Chocolate" you probably were not thinking about just how accurately this food is named while you took each bite! But, even if you did and you vowed to eat "low-fat" or "fat-free" alternatives instead, I have really sad news for you. Since Americans became obsessed with the idea of eating a low-fat diet nearly 30 years ago, we actually have become fatter than ever! We also have become sicker than ever!

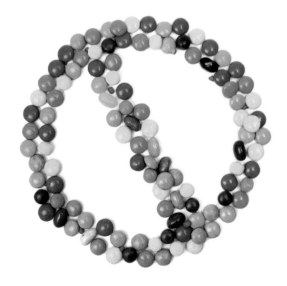

In this time, we have seen an alarming rise in the incidence of stroke, heart disease, liver disease, and diabetes . . . including juvenile diabetes. How has this happened?

When the American Heart Association began the campaign to decrease fat in the American diet, Madison Avenue saw the opportunity and jumped on the bandwagon. The era of "Fat-Free Foods" was born. Unfortunately, fat-free foods tasted, at best, like warmed-over recycled food, and, at worst, like cardboard. Food manufacturers then figured out that they could make low-fat and fat-free foods palatable if they added enough sugar and salt.

Even worse, the food manufacturers learned that high fructose corn syrup (HFCS) is both cost-effective and able to make low-fat and fat-free foods retain the properties that most closely resemble their fat-filled cousins. If you take the time to read the labels of most of the processed foods you touch in the grocery store, you likely will be surprised at some of the foods that contain HFCS. It seems that it is in nearly everything . . . including processed meats and nearly all breads, cereals, condiments, crackers, popcorn, and other processed foods. Many fast food restaurants even add HFCS to their hamburgers!

But, if adding HFCS means that our foods are now fat free or low fat, why are we getting fatter and sicker than ever? To understand why, we must first understand the physiological effects of sugar on the body.

"But isn't fructose the sugar from fruit? That should be good for me . . . right?"

Actually, too much sugar of any kind is detrimental to your health. But here are a few facts about fructose:

The Damaging Effects of too Much "UNWRAPPED" Fructose:

- Insulin resistance
- Obesity
- Metabolic Syndrome (making it extremely difficult to lose weight, even when dieting)
- High triglycerides
- High cholesterol (especially the bad one, LDL)
- Uric acid formation (which leads to hypertension and gout)
- Non-alcoholic fatty liver

Fructose also speeds up aging through a process known as "Advanced Glycation End products" or AGEs. To understand this process, picture the way that sugar browns as it is heated. Fructose does the same thing in your body! Fructose forms AGEs seven times faster than glucose. These AGEs stick to proteins in your body and cause atherosclerosis and even wrinkles! So, if you want to avoid plastic surgery, avoid fructose!

For a great education about fructose metabolism, watch Dr. Robert Lustig's lecture "The Bitter Truth" on YouTube.

"If fructose is bad, then why is fruit good for me?"
"When God made the poison, he packaged it with the antidote."
- Robert Lustig, MD

- Fruit is perfectly packaged in fiber, which slows absorption and contains enzymes to aid in the digestive process.

- Fruit should be eaten in moderation, as it is still a high-sugar food, but the high-fiber, water-rich composition of fruit makes it a healthy choice. The American diet is pathetically lacking in fiber.

- Fruit is loaded with phytonutrients, micronutrients, vitamins, and antioxidants.

- Fruit is not "processed" with cheap oils or other man-made fillers.

- Fruit doesn't create insulin resistance and food addiction. How many "fruit addicts" do you know? Have you ever binged on apples? But fruit still should be eaten in moderation.

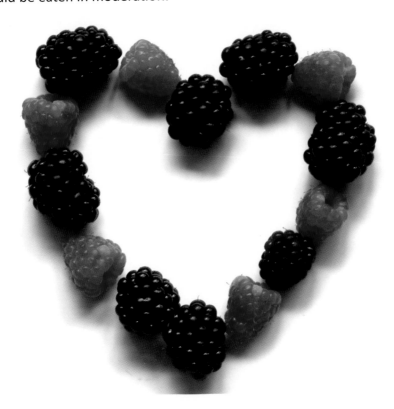

NERD NOTE!

The Glycemic Index (GI) and the Glycemic Load (GL)

The Glycemic Index is a way to measure how fast a certain carbohydrate will raise your blood sugar. The higher a carbohydrate is ranked on the Glycemic Index chart, the faster that food is said to raise your blood sugar. The GI of a carbohydrate is affected by the amount of fiber, fat, and protein in the food. Fiber, fat, and protein slow down the glycemic effect of carbohydrates. This is why it is thought to be very important to choose to eat fruits high in fiber. This is also why vegetables are the healthiest carbohydrates available.

While the Glycemic Index is a way to measure how fast a certain carbohydrate will raise your blood sugar, the Glycemic Load refers to the ranking system for carbohydrate content in food portions that is based on their GI and their portion size. The GL of a carbohydrate combines the quality and the quantity of a carbohydrate into one number. Therefore, GL gives a more accurate picture of what happens when you eat a certain amount of a certain carbohydrate. In other words, eating a smaller portion of a food with a high GI will not raise your blood sugar as much as eating twice as much of the same food.

While it remains important to decrease the overall GI of the carbohydrates you consume, especially if you are consuming them individually, you can control the GL of a meal by eating a combination of high-quality lean proteins, fiber, and healthy fats along with the carbohydrates. This means that you can manipulate the GL of a meal, to some degree, according to the amount of fat and protein you add to your meal. No matter what though, avoid eating carbs that raise your blood sugar quickly by themselves, especially if they have a high GI.

See Appendix 1 for a Glycemic Index Rating of Common Foods.

Now that you know about high fructose corn syrup and fruit, you may be wondering about the myriad of other sweeteners on the market. There is a lot of bad news, but there is some hope as well!

The Bittersweet Facts About Artificial Sweeteners

Artificial sweeteners are not healthy substitutes for sweetening your favorite drinks. They are calorie free, but they offer little in exchange for the risk they present. Nearly all artificial sweeteners have seen their share of controversy . . . and this is not without good reason. We now have evidence that artificial sweeteners elevate insulin levels because they send a signal to the brain that "something sweet is coming." Many of them convert to ethanol in the system. Some are processed with chlorine. So, eliminate these artificial sweeteners as much as possible!

Saccharine (Sweet'N Low): Made through the chemical reaction of anthranilic acid, nitrous oxide, sulfur dioxide, chlorine, and ammonia. In the 1970s studies linked saccharine to bladder cancer. In 2000, it was determined that the connection between bladder cancer in rats and saccharine was not associated to humans. The controversy continues.

Aspartame (NutraSweet): When aspartame is heated or in an unstable environment, it breaks down to phenylalanine, aspartic acid, and methanol! In certain environments, aspartame is shown to break down further to formaldehyde and formic acid. Aspartame has a pH of 4.3, which is very acidic. (The pH scales ranges from 0-14, with 7 considered to be neutral. Numbers below 7 are more acidic; numbers above 7 are more alkaline.) It is not a good choice for cooking, as it begins decomposing at 180 degrees F. For an excellent education about the health effects of aspartame, check out Dr. Mercola's website, www.mercola.com.

Sucralose (Splenda): Probably the most popular artificial sweetener used today, it is 600 times sweeter than sugar, but it is derived from sugar. It is produced by chlorinating sugar (this is a simplified explanation). Like all other artificial sweeteners, sucralose has seen its share of controversy. While the FDA has determined that it is safe for human consumption, there has been some concern about the effect of sucralose on the thymus and the possibility that it decreases the amount of good bacteria in the intestines, while increasing the pH. These studies, conducted on rats, haven't been linked to humans at this time.

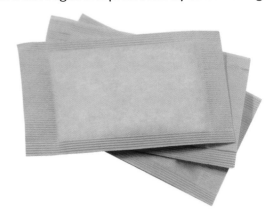

Sugars by Any Other Name

Sucrose, or table sugar, is a lousy choice as a sweetener because of the effect it has on blood sugar. It spikes blood sugar and causes a rapid release of insulin. Sucrose is half glucose and half fructose . . . and fructose is poisonous to the liver.

Honey is not much different from table sugar in regard to the effect that it has on blood sugar, but it does seem to have other minimal health benefits that are not seen with table sugar. Like table sugar, it is nearly equal parts fructose and glucose, but almost 18 percent of honey is made up of water. It also contains trace amounts of vitamins and minerals and small amounts of antioxidants. I prefer unfiltered, un-pasteurized honey because pasteurization kills any live enzymes and nutritional benefits that honey may have. So, raw honey is a good option as a natural sweetener, but it should be used in very minimal amounts. In fact, honey's main claim to fame is the anti-inflammatory and anti-bacterial properties that it has shown is some studies. Its best use is as a topical wound treatment! ***And remember, honey should never be given to children under the age of one year due to the risk of contracting botulism.***

Agave nectar, extracted from the agave plant, is sweeter than honey. It varies in composition depending upon its source, but it generally is said to be **80-90 percent fructose** and 10-20 percent glucose. I was saddened to learn this since agave used to be one of my favorite sweeteners for cooking. But this high fructose content also means that agave is advertised as being "the best" sweetener for diabetics. Since fructose doesn't cause the same insulin spike reaction as sucrose, it is referred to as a "low-glycemic sweetener." But fructose is more toxic to the liver and ultimately leads to Metabolic Syndrome, fatty liver, and insulin resistance! Like all sugars, agave should be used in very small amounts.

Pure maple syrup, like honey and table sugar, is nearly equal parts fructose and glucose. It is also 18-20 percent water. Maple syrup has trace minerals and actually has significant amounts of zinc and manganese. But use caution when purchasing maple syrup. Since it is expensive to manufacture, many companies have figured out cheap ways to capitalize on this tasty syrup. Most "pancake" syrups have no maple in them at all! If you read the ingredients, they are primarily made of high fructose corn syrup and artificial flavoring. Not only do they lack pure maple syrup's minimal health benefits, but they are truly atrocious for your health! Artificial maple syrup should not be used at all and pure maple syrup should be used, like all sugars, in minimal amounts. But, pure maple syrup is preferable to table sugar.

The "Skinny" on Other Sweeteners

Sugar alcohols such as maltitol, erythritol, and xylitol might sound like the perfect combination of your favorite wine and chocolate, but they are not alcohol at all, and they won't get you drunk! They obtained the name "sugar alcohols" because their chemical structure resembles half of a sugar molecule and half of an alcohol molecule. They are naturally occurring in many plants and berries.

The good news is that they are very effective sweeteners and a good alternative for diabetics and people who are insulin resistant. Since it's very difficult for the body to digest sugar alcohols, they stay in the digestive tract much longer than sugar. In turn, they do not cause the same insulin spikes that sugar causes so the insulin release is much slower.

But be wary even with the good news about sugar alcohols. They are not calorie free or sugar free (as marketing experts would have you believe), though they do count anywhere from 30-50 percent less than sugar, and they don't figure into actual sugar grams. Instead, they are separated into their own category as "sugar alcohols" and they figure into the total carbohydrate tally. So, if something has 10g of sugar alcohols, it counts as 5g of carbohydrates.

There is also bad news about sugar alcohols. Since they are so hard for the body to digest, they sit in the digestive tract for an extended period of time. This leads to fermentation . . . Yikes! How do you spell relief? In small amounts sugar alcohols don't usually cause much of a problem. But, in excess, they can cause serious bloating, cramps, flatulence, and diarrhea.

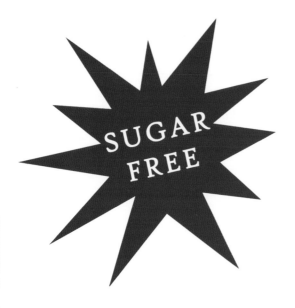

But, the worst news about sugar alcohols is associated with the marketing. Since they are not technically sugar, manufacturers can advertise foods containing them as "sugar free." This is very misleading, especially for diabetics and people who are insulin resistant. Consuming foods with sugar alcohols is much better than consuming sugar, but not knowing your total carb load or believing that you are consuming "sugar-free" foods can be a major problem.

Use Stevia in Place of Sugar

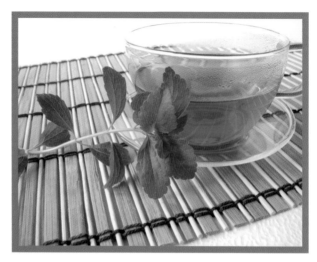

Stevia, extracted from the Stevia leaf, is my favorite sweetener. It is processed by drying out Stevia leaves through a water extraction process and it is refined using ethanol, methanol, and crystallization. It then goes through ultrafiltration and nanofiltration. *You do need to be careful that the brand you purchase does not contain alcohol, though!*

Also, I am aware that early testing did show some concern that Stevia may be genotoxic. However, it was determined that the data from the testing was mishandled. Further studies have determined that Stevia is not genotoxic and that it shows no signs of being carcinogenic or of causing birth defects. On the contrary, Stevia has been shown to have many health benefits. *It does not alter blood sugar in measurable amounts, and current medical research shows promising evidence that Stevia has a positive effect on hypertension!*

NERD NOTE!
Insulin Resistance:

"Help! I'm Drowning in Sugar and I Can't Get Out!"

Chronic, excessive sugar consumption, no matter its form, can lead to *hyperinsulinemia.* All carbohydrates must be broken down to their simplest form, monosaccharides (glucose and fructose - for the sake of simplicity), before they enter the bloodstream and can be used for energy. It doesn't matter if it is licorice, pasta, brown rice, or oatmeal; it must be broken down to its tiniest building blocks . . . sugar. Once the blood sugar is elevated, insulin is released in an attempt to push glucose into our cells.

It's important to have just enough glucose for energy, but not too much. If you overdose your system with simple carbs (aka sugar), you keep your body in a chronic state of hyperinsulinemia. Once the liver and muscle cells are full of sugar, the excess carbs are converted to a fat called palmitic acid (PA). PA seriously interferes with the hormonal response and sensitivity to leptin (the hormone released in the gut that tells your brain you are full).

At this point the insulin can't push any more glucose into the liver, and the liver and your muscles become "insulin resistant." Your glucose level continues to go higher and higher because there is nowhere for it to be stored, and your body is not getting the signal that the cells are full while the insulin is present in your blood. All the while, your body thinks it needs more glucose because of the presence of insulin, and you start craving carbs! Eventually, the liver is totally overwhelmed and all the fat that is being created to deal with the excess sugar can no longer be sent into systemic circulation so it gets stored in the liver. That's right, you get fatty liver, just like an alcoholic!

This is bad enough, but it isn't even close to the end of the picture. The hormone cortisol comes to the "rescue" because your body doesn't like the perceived "low blood sugar" it senses (even though you are totally drowning in sugar). The cortisol begins converting protein into sugar . . . from your own muscles! This process is called gluconeogenesis. This muscle-wasting process leads to excess fat being deposited around the visceral organs (your gut). When you see people with "muffin tops" (that excess fluff around the middle), it is almost always a sign of excess cortisol, which is almost always a sign of excess carbohydrate consumption and insulin resistance.

This insulin resistance in the fat cells causes the body to be unable to process circulating fatty acids. When this happens, there is increased hydrolysis of stored triglycerides and elevated levels of fatty acids in the blood and you end up with high triglycerides on your blood test. So, in case you aren't following me, I am telling you that high triglycerides are an indication that you are consuming an excessive amount of sugars/simple carbohydrates!

What is so bad about this? Well, with insulin resistance and chronically elevated glucose levels, the pancreas must continue to produce more insulin to compensate . . . until it simply cannot keep up any longer. This is the beginning of Type 2 Diabetes. Aggressive lifestyle modification usually can alter or reverse many of the symptoms of Type 2 Diabetes, but only to a point. Eventually the burden on your body will be too great.

For the final touch, the pancreatic beta cells, which have already taken massive abuse from the overproduction of insulin, are further affected by the highly destructive, oxidative process that occurs when sugar sticks to protein. These pesky complexes, referred to as "Advanced Glycated End products" (AGEs), become oxidized and lead to rapid aging. Since the pancreas has been highly compromised, it is one of the most vulnerable organs when it comes to AGEs. With enough abuse, the beta cells will become permanently damaged, just like they are in people who suffer from Type 1 Diabetes. Your life will never be the same!

I hope this is getting your attention. While it's never too late to start making positive changes, the sooner you start the better. Eventually your body will not be able to effectively fight the ravaging effects of the years of bad choices. Once your organs start deteriorating, they usually start doing so in rapid succession. Diseases like diabetes, cancer, and heart disease are devastating to overall health and well being. The timer is set differently for everyone depending upon genetics, environmental influences, and the degree of abuse, but do know: Chronically elevated blood insulin and obesity are associated with systemic inflammation and many types of cancer. *In case this is still unclear, excess sugar and simple carbs will kill you early!*

Fight Insulin Resistance!

- Get the majority of your carb consumption from vegetables and a little from fruit.

- The fiber, micronutrients, and phytonutrients in vegetables make them a great source of carbohydrates. They digest slowly and provide far more nutrition than the amount of glucose they provide . . . especially greens!

- It becomes virtually impossible to burn fat with chronically elevated insulin levels.

- Elevated blood insulin ultimately causes distortions in hunger/satiety hormone signaling.

- Chronic sugar/carb consumption makes you think you are hungry even though you may have just eaten.

- There is very little nutritional value (micronutrients and phytonutrients) in grains for the amount of sugar they provide. Eat them sparingly!

So, it is very clear now that the consumption of the wrong sugars is toxic to your body, and it is very clear now that the excessive consumption of all sugars is really toxic to your body. But there are a few other foods that you may be very surprised to learn are toxic to your body as well—milk, soy, genetically modified foods and oils—even the "good" ones.

Does Milk Build Strong Bones?

If you bought this book as a companion to the *Eat healthy With the Brain Doctor's Wife Cookbook*, then you may have noticed that none of the recipes in our cookbook call for milk or any other dairy products. We use almond milk or rice milk in place of dairy milk, and we use nuts or other wholesome choices in place of cheese. While it is not my objective to destroy your love of dairy products, you should know a few simple facts.

- Mammals are not designed to drink milk past infancy.

- Humans are genetically coded to become intolerant to lactase (the enzyme that digests lactose) once we are about 2 years old. Only about ⅓ of the world's population remains able to effectively digest lactose beyond infancy.

- Lactose is broken down into galactose and glucose (if you are not lactose intolerant), which elevates blood sugar.

- While the government and the dairy industry urge people to drink at least three glasses of milk every day, nutrition experts from Harvard and Cornell believe that amount is way over the top.

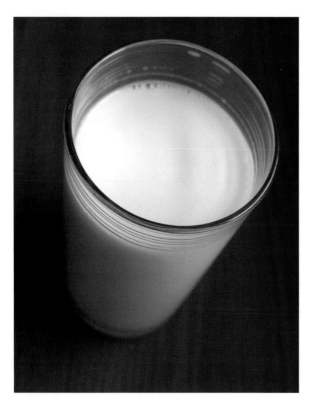

- Studies have shown that the high level of calcium in milk IS NOT easily utilized by the body and does not improve bone strength.

- There is no evidence that a diet high in calcium increases bone strength. Many studies have shown the opposite!

- Green, leafy vegetables, vitamin D, exercise, and increased protein intake are far more effective ways to increase the assimilation of calcium.

NERD NOTE!
Why Milk Does NOT Do a Body Good!

In addition to all of the reasons listed above, pasteurization – the process of heating milk to high temperatures for a short time to kill bacteria — also kills most of the live enzymes that may have made milk worth drinking. While pasteurization is a necessary process in our culture, it renders milk relatively useless, nutritionally speaking. Furthermore, homogenization, the process of pumping milk through small tubules to break up fat globules so that the fat does not separate from the milk, may have an increased relationship to arteriosclerosis due to the breakdown of plasminogen during this process.

But, one of the most disturbing aspects of milk processing comes from the fairly recent introduction of the bovine growth hormones rBST and rBGH to milk. rBST and rBGH commonly are given to dairy cows to increase milk production. Their presence in the milk you drink stimulates the production of IGF-1 (insulin growth factor) by your liver. Milk already contains a significant amount of IGF-1, but the addition of these hormones causes your body to produce even more! *IGF-1 is necessary for growth — in the right amounts and at the right times — but excessive IGF-1 has been strongly correlated with breast, colon, and prostate cancer.*

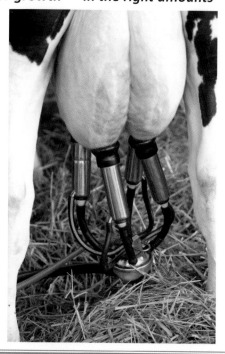

rBGH supplement also increases the rates of mastitis and infections in dairy cows. These find their way into your milk. This is why dairy cows are treated with antibiotics . . . which also find their way into your milk. Ultimately, this could lead to antibiotic-resistant bacterial infections in the environment. So, although America widely uses rBGH supplements for dairy cows, many other countries have banned milk from cows that have been treated with rBGH.

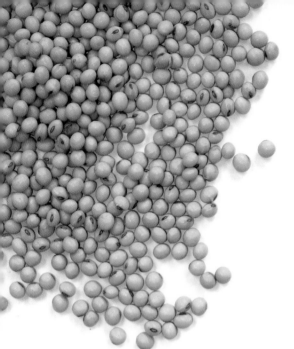

Soy

I would love to tell you that soy is the miracle food for replacing dairy, but this hasn't turned out to be the case. There does seem to be many health benefits related to the moderate consumption of soybeans (unless you are sensitive to lectins!) and vegetarians may find it necessary to consume a little tofu, but excessive amounts of soy products have been shown to cause multiple health issues.

- Soy is highly concentrated with lectins (we will talk more about this later).

- Soy contains high levels of omega-6 fatty acids. Some omega-6 fatty acids are essential for the production of arachadonic acid (which affects the inflammatory response). But, in excess, this can lead to systemic inflammation. The key is to balance the omega-3/omega-6 fatty acid ratio, but doing so is a major problem among Americans.

- Soy products are so inexpensive to produce that soy oil and proteins are widely used in processed food. This elevates the consumption of omega-6 fatty acids beyond the healthy limit.

- **Soy protein in soy milk has been shown to cause the liver to produce as much IGF-1 as dairy milk does, if not more!**

- Soy contains isoflavones. The isoflavones genistein and daizein are a source of phytoestrogens. These ultimately bind to estrogen receptor sites. Some experts claim that these help to prevent cancer, while others claim that these same isoflavones actually cause cancer.

- Phytoestrogens may be responsible for early puberty in young females and for impotence in men.

- Soybeans also contain a high level of phytic acid, a known chelating agent, antioxidant, and anti-inflammatory agent. Since phytic acid has a chelating effect, it is blamed for reducing the absorption of vital minerals.

- The majority of soy crops in the United States are genetically modified. The number has been estimated at 70 percent and as high as 97 percent.

Genetically Modified (GM) Foods:
What are they and why are they so controversial?

- GM foods have had their DNA altered in some way through genetic engineering.

- GM crops are bred to be pest and/or herbicide resistant, to be heartier and more able to withstand extreme conditions, to have faster growth rates, etc.

- Scientists can make nearly any desired change to GM foods by isolating certain chromosomes.

- GM foods have been marketed in stores for just over a decade. This does not give us a clear picture of the long term effects of genetically modified organisms (GMOs) on humans.

- Humans have been experiencing a host of health issues, including increasing rates of disease and allergies, for the past decade. There is no effective or easy way to test if the effects of GMOs are responsible.

- Once the FDA determines that a GMO is safe for human consumption, food manufacturers are not required to label foods as "genetically modified." This means that you lose the ability to choose!

- America leads the race in GMOs by nearly three times more than any other country. This includes about 90 percent of soy crops, with corn and cotton crops close behind.

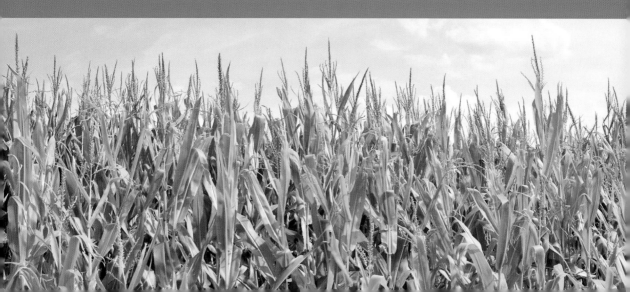

GMOs

Genetically Modified foods have had their DNA altered in some way through genetic engineering. In the case of produce, this is very different from traditional plant breeding in which breeders use a variety of techniques, including in vitro techniques, to create a hybrid plant from two plants or crops that are related. An example of this would be like breeding two types of dogs; they are from the same species, just different breeds. GM techniques involve the actual alteration or modification of the DNA of plants or crops through the insertion or deletion of a certain gene into the chosen plant. GM foods have been marketed in stores for just over a decade. There are a host of reasons

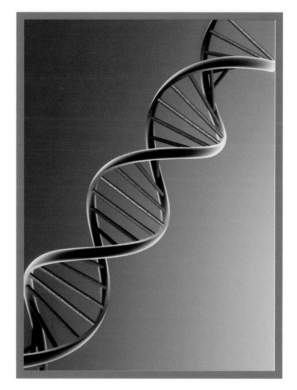

that food manufactures have embarked on this relatively new, experimental task. A wide variety of alterations can be made to foods, which seems desirable upon first inspection. Crops can be bred to be pest resistant, herbicide resistant, heartier, and more able to withstand extreme conditions, faster growth rates, etc. Scientists can make nearly any desired change they choose by isolating certain chromosomes.

However, the FDA does not have clear and specific methods for testing GM foods. Rather, they review data submitted by manufacturers of the foods. They simply acknowledge that the creators of the GM foods who have submitted the data claim that they have tested the new creation and that it is safe for consumption. There are many books written about the inadequate or misleading studies done on GM foods. In the book *Genetic Roulette*, Jeffrey M. Smith writes a detailed description, as well as insider documents, of GMO safety trials and the health risks and complications associated to specific GM crops.

Of the risks and complications associated with GM foods, the one I find the most disturbing is that food companies are not required to label foods that have been modified once the FDA has determined that they are safe for human consumption. Many people would boycott foods that they knew were GM. In reality, nearly 90 percent of the soybeans consumed in America come from GM crops with corn and cotton closely following. America leads the pack in genetic modification of foods by nearly three times any other country.

While ag biotech companies would have you think that there are no risks associated with consuming GM foods because we have been consuming them in mass quantities for well over a decade, that is misleading at best. The truth is, we have no way of really knowing if the rise in many diseases we have seen over the past 10 years may be related to genetic modification. In fact there are many risks associated with genetic modification, mutagenesis, and the techniques required to accomplish the end result. But we are told little of these risks, only of the great "potential" benefits.

Understanding the deep and long-term effects that GM foods have had or are just beginning to have would require a massive undertaking. It would require epidemiological studies to be conducted on populations of people who consume GM foods over long periods of time. Without those studies it is virtually impossible to determine the effects of GM foods on the public. It is also likely that the Biotech companies understand how difficult it would be to ever show the connection between GM foods and the rash of new allergies and health crises that have been occurring over the past decade.

It is a personal decision whether or not to purchase organic produce, which has not been genetically altered. If you are comfortable with the idea of GM foods, they

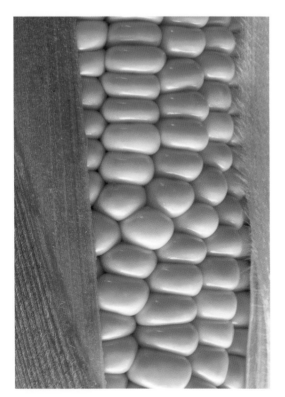

are certainly more affordable. But you deserve to know what you are eating. Your health is your responsibility. Without a healthy brain and a healthy body, you can't be your best in life.

Let's Get an Oil Check

I am just going to start by saying that you should never purchase cheap vegetable oils that are high in omega-6 fatty acids such as corn oil, safflower oil, and soy-based oils. Also, when you do purchase ANY oil, make certain that its color resembles the oil's natural source. Nut oils should be dark or a deep gold. Olive oils should be a deep, dark greenish color. Coconut oil should be white. There is still a lot more for you to consider when it comes to oils, though.

Cooking Oils

While there are many oils that are very healthy for consumption, there are few that are healthy when you use them for cooking. Oils become toxic when they reach their smoking point during cooking. For most oils, this occurs at a relatively low temperature. Some of the oils that are best for cooking at low temperatures are avocado, walnut, almond, and grape seed. Most of these oils are easily found at your local health food store but may not be so easily found at the corner grocery store. For cooking at temperatures that are over the medium-high heat setting, I remain an advocate of oils that are solid at room temperature such as organic butter, ghee, or coconut oil. No matter what oil I choose to cook with, though, I make sure to use it sparingly! I prefer getting my healthy fats by eating them in natural form or by using uncooked oils on salad.

Coconut Oil

There continues to be a lot of debate over the benefits and supposed risks of coconut oil. Some experts claim that it is a health food that promotes weight loss and lowers cholesterol, while others say that coconut oil causes weight gain and high cholesterol. However, it appears that most of the outdated studies that condemned coconut oil were using "hydrogenated" versions of coconut oil. Hydrogenation is a process that creates "trans fats."

In its natural form, coconut oil is a saturated fat. However, it is a plant-based fat, not an animal-based fat like butter. It is also a medium-chain triglyceride, or fatty acid, as opposed to a long-chain fatty acid, like animal fats. There is a huge difference in the way your body assimilates these fats. Small- and medium-chain fatty acids, such as coconut oil, are digested and absorbed immediately through the liver and are quickly available for energy. This makes them less likely to cause obesity and high cholesterol. In addition, coconut oil also has been shown to have many anti-viral and anti-fungal properties.

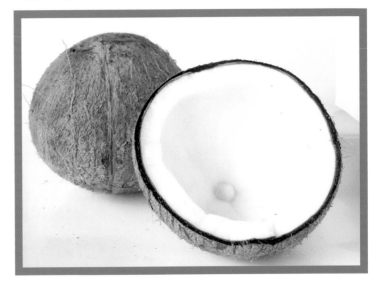

Canola Oil

I am not inclined to tell you that you should or shouldn't use canola oil, but I would like to shed some light on the controversy surrounding canola oil so that you can make an informed decision.

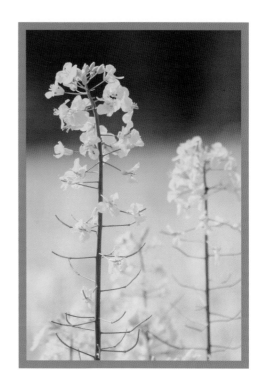

Have you ever seen canola growing in the wild? Have you ever picked up some fresh canola from the grocery store? I didn't think so! Canola is a made up name that is derived from the words, "Canada, Low Acid, and Oil." The "canola" plant is the product of plant breeding so we often hear that canola is a "genetically modified organism," or GMO. Technically that would be true since the plant came into existence as a result of traditional plant breeding. But the story behind Canola goes deeper...

So why was canola developed? Canola is bred from the rapeseed plant. Rapeseed plants have long been used for their oil. However, rapeseed oil has been used primarily for industrial purposes. In fact, it makes an excellent lubricant for machinery! But, rapeseed oil also has been used in small amounts by many cultures for thousands of years for cooking. However, we now know that rapeseed oil is toxic when it is used for cooking if it is not used in small amounts. As cooking oil, rapeseed oil has been linked to lung cancer and myocardial lesions.

In addition, rapeseed oil is high in erucic acid (which only has some health benefits when it is consumed in its natural form) and in glucosinolates (which give it a bitter taste). So, in an attempt to make this easily obtainable oil into a more consumable oil, plant breeders in Canada worked until they created a plant that could be turned into an oil that the FDA would accept — the "canola." During this process, they ended up with oil that is primarily a monounsaturated fat, which is a good thing; but that is also high in omega-6 fatty acids, which is not a good thing.

However, since 1998, more and more of the "canola" plants have been further genetically engineered to create a more herbicide-resistant plant. So, now you have a plant that was created by cross-breeding plants to obtain a plant healthy enough for human consumption and you are further genetically modifying it to resist herbicides and bugs!

The FDA has determined that canola is healthy for human consumption. They say the same thing about Coca-Cola, high fructose corn syrup, and a myriad of genetically modified organisms. So if you trust the FDA to tell you what is healthy for human consumption, go for it. But beware! Just because something is fit for human consumption does not mean that it is optimal for human health! I personally prefer to avoid substances shrouded in this much controversy. When there are so many wholesome choices available, why take chances with one that is uncertain? And if you are going to purchase canola oil, make sure that it is organic.

NERD NOTE!
Processing Oils

You may have noticed that most oils in the grocery store are light in color and are packaged in clear plastic bottles. Yet, most oils are naturally dark in color or resemble the color of the source they came from. And, more than that, the natural, dark color of most oils attracts light, which will destroy the oil and quickly turn it rancid unless it is stored in dark, light-repellent bottles or in refrigerators. So, how do those gleaming shelves of light-colored, highly-visible oils get filled?

First of all, marketing companies long ago discovered that consumers are more drawn to lighter-colored oils that they can see through clear bottles. In addition, manufacturers learned that cooking oils are less expensive and available in greater quantities when they are processed by chemical extraction. In this process, hexane, or some other form of petroleum solvent, separates the oil from its natural nut, seed, or plant. The resulting oil is then bleached and deodorized to remove the natural color and odor. But the oil is not ready to be sold yet! Since chemical processing leaves traces of petroleum-based products, the oil is then boiled to remove the undesirable by-products of processing. Preservatives are added to extend shelf life. The result is "oil" that in no way resembles its natural origins and has very little nutritional value.

If this does not sit well with you, there is an option. You can purchase expeller-pressed oils or cold-pressed oils. These processes also have their limitations; however, they are significantly better than chemical extraction processing. Since these oils usually do not contain any kind of preservative, they generally are bottled in dark plastic or glass bottles to preserve their shelf life. For this same reason, it is highly recommended that you refrigerate your oil after opening, especially if you don't consume it quickly.

These oils do tend to be more expensive and usually must be purchased from health food and gourmet stores so they are not as "convenient" or "cost-effective" as the mass-produced grocery store varieties. You have to decide how important this issue is in relation to your health. For me, and the health of my family, it's a "big brainer."

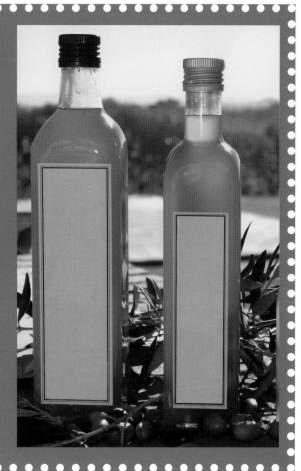

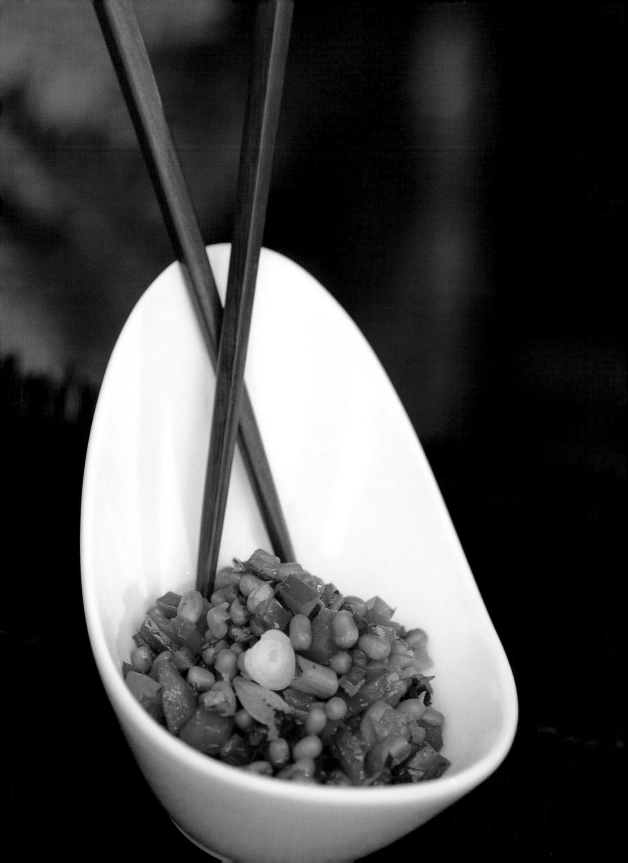

Chapter 3
GOING FROM LETHAL TO LUSCIOUS!

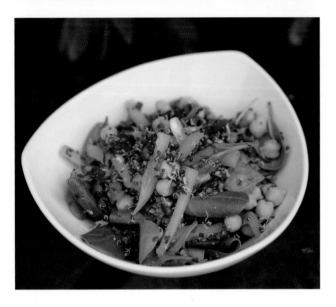

How is your relationship with food? Are you tantalizing your palate with luscious, life-giving foods from the "rainbow" like organic salads with grilled salmon and "Brain Balancing Smoothies?" Or, are you poisoning your body with foods that you've been told are healthy? Are you bankrupting your energy and toxifying your cells with lethal processed foods, fast foods, and inflammation-causing sugars?

If you answered "Yes" to the last two questions, you are not alone. We all have been bamboozled! If you are addicted to the major toxins that age our bodies and destroy our health, it's not your fault! Our society is inundated with anti-nutrition, genetically modified, sugar-filled, and inflammation-causing foods. These foods are disguised by a multitude of names, and the food manufacturers and bioengineers don't want you to know the truth! As a society, we have distorted everything about food. Some people actually believe that fried zucchini counts as a serving of vegetables and potato chips are a real form of potatoes!

NERD NOTE!
[Adult Baby Food Anyone?]

Nearly all food items in most fast-food restaurants contain added sugar, high fructose corn syrup, salt, and cheap oil such as corn, safflower, or soy oil. This includes the hamburger meat and the buns! Also, the fiber and the gristle are removed from many fast foods. This might be forgivable and easy to understand if the only reason for this was to extend shelf life and make shipping possible.

However, the reason for all this processing is much more devious than you may think.

Believe it or not, there are actually "food consultants." These people should have to wear a permanent tattoo that reads "anti-nutrition consultants!" It is their job to discover what drives human behavior and to come up with the combinations of foods that activate the opiate and dopamine centers in the human brain . . . and they have succeeded! They discovered that the right combination of salt, fat, and sugar will act similarly to heroin or cocaine on the opiate centers in your brain. This makes you totally addicted to food that comes in those combinations! More than that, these "consultants" come up with new ideas for "food" that will cause you to unconsciously choose one brand over another.

Even more insidiously, the "food consultants" also know how to make you want more of those foods! The combination of excessive fat (especially omega-6 fatty acids like corn, soy, and safflower oil), sugar, and salt hijack the signal of the hunger/satiety hormones in your body. The result is that you don't feel satisfied even after you have gorged. You may feel uncomfortable around the waistline, but your brain doesn't know you are full and it wants more! "Bet you can't eat just one!"

These "consultants" also discovered that there is a link between the feelings of pleasure and decreased chewing time. As a result, fiber and gristle are removed from foods and replaced with even more fat. The resulting "food" product hardly needs to be chewed; it just sort of slides down your throat like baby food!

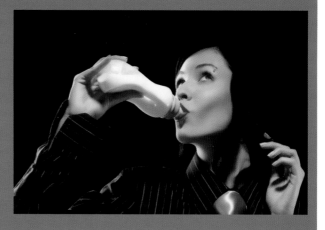

For a more in-depth look behind the scenes of the fast-food industry, Dr. David Kessler gives a frighteningly descriptive account in his book *The End of Overeating*.

Going Against the Grain!

Sadly, our society also is inundated with misinformation about "healthy" foods like whole grains, legumes, juices, and even those "healthy" fast-food options. This may be one of the greatest challenges that we face in our quest to live a truly healthy life!

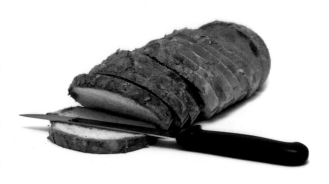

I have been affected deeply by this kind of misinformation. For years I was a "pescatarian," adhering to a nearly vegan diet of no dairy and no meat other than a little, occasional deep-sea fish. I ate a "wholesome" diet rich with vegetables, fruit, nuts, seeds, and LOTS of grains, rice, whole grain breads, and quinoa. I thought my diet was perfect . . . until I went in for my checkup.

As I mentioned earlier, I was 118 pounds and had 13 percent body fat, but my cholesterol was 260 and my triglycerides were over 300! I also was insulin resistant and had Polycystic Ovarian Syndrome. This made no sense because I had adopted this diet after having my gall bladder removed and after being told that I was eating too much fat and cholesterol. As a "pescatarian," I was eating a low-fat diet that was virtually cholesterol free! Yet, my blood work indicated that I was getting sicker on the inside, not better. So now what was the problem? Back to the research room for me!

It turns out that my much-loved grains did not love me! And it went even further. I had a food sensitivity test performed which showed significant reactions to most grains, legumes, dairy, soy, and gluten. I also discovered that I am not alone. Gluten, saponins, and lectins, which are found in grains, dairy products, and some vegetables, are problematic for digestion in many, if not most, people.

A Note About Gluten . . .

Gluten is a hot topic these days so you already may have heard about gluten sensitivities. You may even know someone who has to eat a gluten-free diet. But what does this really mean? Gluten is a sticky protein substance found in wheat, barley, rye, and many other grains. It is in virtually all foods that contain flour, unless it is otherwise specified. Also, gluten sensitivity is far more common than you may realize. More than 3 million Americans suffer from the effects of gluten sensitivity and 99 percent of people don't even know it! Gluten can increase the permeability of the intestinal lining, and symptoms of gluten sensitivities include Celiac Sprue and Crohn's disease, rheumatoid arthritis, cancer, obesity, allergies, heart disease, osteoporosis, anemia, fatigue, multiple sclerosis, depression, dementia, migraines, and most other autoimmune disorders.

Unlike gluten, though, not much is espoused about saponins and lectins. Saponins are what soap is made of, and they are found in soy and in many grains and legumes. While their antifungal, antibacterial properties make them great detergents, they can cause damage to our intestines and they can prevent the absorption of nutrients in our systems.

Lectins, likewise, are in many of the foods we eat and can be very harmful to our health. In fact, most foods contain lectins, but some foods, such as wheat, rice, oats, buckwheat, millet, rye, corn, quinoa, dairy, legumes, soy, eggplant, potatoes, and tomatoes, contain high concentrations of lectins. This can prove to be toxic and can lead to many health issues including insulin resistance.

The story goes something like this: Lectins are tough, exterior, sugar-binding proteins on many plants. When they are consumed, they are resistant to digestive enzymes and acids. They also bind themselves to the microvilli in the intestines and damage the intestinal walls. This makes lectins a great natural pesticide for grains and other plants.

For the human digestive system, this means that lectins are not broken down into

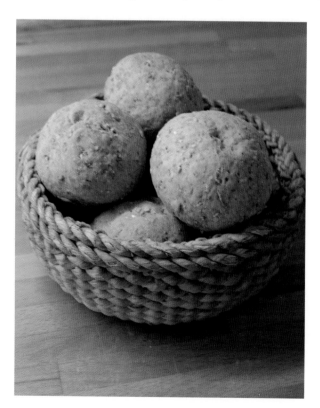

their basic building blocks, amino acids. Through a complex chemical process, which increases the permeability of the intestinal lining (basically, the cells don't hold together tightly), "leaky gut" occurs and lectins pass through the damaged intestinal lining as whole protein molecules. Since the body is designed to receive "amino acids," it doesn't recognize these large proteins and it triggers an antigen/antibody response to these foreign invaders. This can cause new allergies.

Also, since lectins are carbohydrate-binding proteins, they can bind to unintended carbohydrates within cell membranes where they act like a key opening a lock. As a result, a myriad of undesirable reactions are unleashed such as autoimmune disorders, Crohn's disease, allergies, heart disease, cancer, obesity, migraines, and Polycystic Ovarian Syndrome.

These symptoms are similar to those of patients with gluten sensitivites; however, many people will go to the doctor for testing only to find out that they are not gluten sensitive. These people are not told about lectins, and they often feel so frustrated that they give up on their quest for good health.

If this is the case with you or someone that you know, you may want to try an elimination diet for two weeks. If you eliminate bread, flour, all grains, all legumes, sugar, dairy, soy, tomatoes, potatoes, and eggplant for two weeks, you will be able to determine if you are sensitive to lectins or not. The results will be nearly immediate and they will be dramatic. You also may choose to have an IgG test performed, which shows delayed reaction food sensitivities. Many physicians are now performing these tests, but it is still more common with physicians who practice "functional medicine." In addition, they are performed at the Amen Clinics (www.amenclinics.com) and on the East Coast by Dr. Mark Hyman (www.drhyman.com).

After learning about all of this and realizing that grains and legumes made up about 30 percent of my diet at the time, I found myself in a quandary. But, after recovering from my identity crisis, I decided that my health was more important to me than identifying with a particular diet or lifestyle. So, I ditched the grains and most legumes and I have never felt better! Now, on the rare occasion that I do consume legumes, I make sure that they are fresh, soaked over night, and thoroughly cooked. When it comes to legumes and other vegetables, preparation makes a difference in the concentration and effect of lectins.

There isn't much that I can say about grains, though, except that if you eat them, they should be eaten as "whole," unprocessed grains instead of as bread. And you should

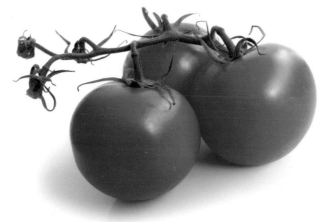

consume them as you would a condiment . . . in very small amounts!

This does not mean that all grains and legumes are "evil" and that no one should eat them. Grains and legumes can be a great source of fiber and protein, especially for vegetarians. Also, not everyone is sensitive to them and certainly not to all of them. But, they definitely are on the "Proceed with Caution" list. They are two of the food categories that are the most problematic on a large scale, and you risk developing sensitivities to them by eating them in excessive amounts. Also, they just don't contain as much nutritional value as fruits and vegetables.

Juices: The Good, the Bad, and the Ugly

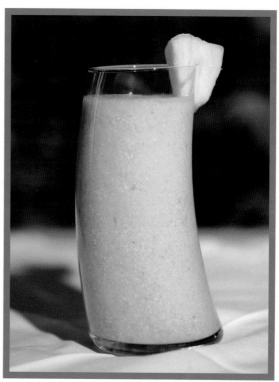

- **Fruit juice**, fresh squeezed or otherwise, should be avoided with few exceptions. Remember, fruit juice is pure fructose with the fiber removed! Other than certain drugs and alcohol, there are few things more toxic to your liver than fructose. The only exceptions are lemon juice and lime juice. They are low-sugar fruits, and adding a little lemon or lime to your water is actually good for you.

- **Fruit smoothies** are better than fruit juice. Blending fruit with water or almond milk, some nuts or seeds, and even some vegetables (I promise you can't taste them!) not only tastes great, but it also gives you a concentrated dose of phytonutrients without leaving the necessary fiber behind. Adding a little protein powder and healthy fat will slow the absorption of the sugar a bit more. Just be careful not to use an excessive amount of fruit. Try to keep it to one piece of fruit or less than one cup of berries.

- **Vegetable juice** is an important food . . . at the right time and for the right reasons.

   First, it's just not possible to eat vegetables all day! Use vegetable juice to supplement your vegetable intake, not to replace eating vegetables!

   Second, when you want quick energy as opposed to needing to digest your food, vegetable juice is a great solution. It doesn't contain the sugar that fruit juice contains and, with the fiber removed, there is no digestion time. As a result, it gives you a quick, concentrated infusion of vitamins, minerals, and phytonutrients. It's like mainlining instant energy and you will be electrocharged! However, vegetable juice should never be a replacement for eating your vegetables. You need the fiber from vegetables!

Third, and maybe most important, the nutrients in vegetables are not as effectively released through chewing and digestion as they are by being mechanically crushed. You would need to eat a whole lot more vegetables to get the same amount of nutrition than you can get in a green drink. And that is exactly what our ancestors did. Without the luxury of the local grocery store and processed foods, their primary foods were vegetables, fruits, berries, nuts, and seeds. They supplemented their diet with protein. The radical change in our lifestyle, affected by industrialization, calls for drastic measures if we don't want to fall victim to the perils of a fast food nation. Vegetable juice is a great start!

- **"Goddess of Greens"** is one of my favorite quick energy "pick me ups." It is a vegetable juice that is made from a combination of kale, celery, cucumber, spinach, parsley, and wheat grass.

- **Wheat grass** is the closest thing humans have to a fountain of youth—as long as you are not allergic. This power-packed elixir contains over 90 minerals and 20 amino acids per ounce, and it is 70 percent chlorophyll. This is terrific news because the chlorophyll molecule is virtually identical to the molecule in hemoglobin.

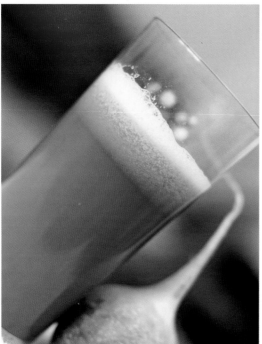

The only difference is that the central atom of hemoglobin is iron and the central atom of wheatgrass is magnesium. As a result, the molecule in wheatgrass juice is quickly absorbed and used for nutrition in the blood. Many pilot studies show that wheat grass has positive effects on increased blood flow, digestion, detoxification, heavy metal chelation, and anti-cancer treatments. Also, wheat grass does not contain gluten since it is a young grass and is cut before the wheat kernel has formed. *However, celiacs should be cautious of the source of their wheat grass and they should consult their physician before deciding to consume wheat grass*.

Fast Foods:

The Few That Don't Contain High Fructose Corn Syrup . . .

- Diet Soda . . . The artificial sweeteners and caffeine do the trick!

- Iced Tea . . . Do you drink it without sugar?

- Coffee . . . I don't even need to explain.

- Milk . . . There are *many* important reasons not to drink milk.

- Chicken Nuggets . . . Many restaurants add dimethylpolysiloxane (an anti-foaming agent) and tertiary butylhydroquinone or TBHQ (a highly toxic chemical preservative). And don't get me started on the "chicken."

- French Fries . . . Do I really need to explain? They are DOUBLE fried in cheap oil and the little bit of potato becomes a refined sugar through this frying process. Then there's the salt. I guess they figured they didn't need HFCS for these. French fries will kill you!

- Hash Browns: It's the same story as French fries.

In a pinch, you can eat . . .

- Baked Potatoes . . . Just don't add the toppings!

- Fruit Cups . . . Don't add yogurt and granola which both contain high fructose corn syrup.

- Salad . . . Only eat the vegetable part. Try salsa instead of dressing. The dressings are loaded with high fructose corn syrup, salt, and fat. And let's not forget the wonderful little candied nuts!

For an enlightening look at how frightening some of these "McFranken-NON-Foods" really are, check out a great article on Dr. Mercola's website at: http://articles.mercola.com/sites/articles/archive/2010/11/08/do-you-have-any-idea-of-the-chemicals-used-in-fast-food-chicken.aspx

So, what do you eat in a world so full of lethal foods? First, you must decide to take your destiny back into your own hands and choose to eat only healthy, luscious foods. You can change your beliefs and educate yourself. Do not allow advertisers, who spend billions of dollars to hypnotically blind you, make your food choices for you. That should infuriate you! Wake up!

Begin this new journey with food by really understanding what you are doing to your body with the foods you have been eating. Educate yourself about all the incredible, healthy, delectable foods that will give you clarity, strength, and energy and even heal your body. Also, don't just cut out the old foods that you think are stealing your health and joy and making you tired (you don't want to feel deprived) . . . add new, amazing foods to your diet. Try new things each day. Make it an adventure to find energizing and healing foods for you and your family.

Also, for the most part, stay out of the center of the grocery stores. As a rule, most of what you need is focused around the outer aisles of the stores. Focus your attention on the produce sections and the fish and meat counters (if you are not a vegetarian). Of course, some of you may need some whole-grain products, some refrigerated products (not ice cream), and spices. But, for Pete's sake, stay away from the potato chips, cookies, and soft drinks!

The food you eat is your best medicine or it is a terrible drug that will take you on a really bad trip!

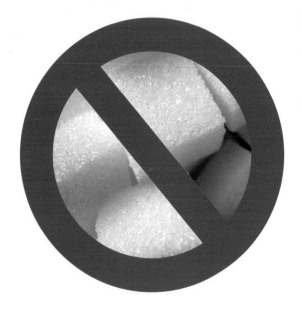

Lethal "Anti-Nutrition"

- Sugar . . . By any other name. It's still sugar and it is poison.

- Vegetables that are breaded and fried . . . Sorry but they don't count!

- Sugar coated and/or cooked fruits

- Fruit juices . . . Yes, even "organic, no sugar added" juice. If the fiber has been removed, you are left with nothing but fructose . . . Not good!

- Dried fruit that is sugar coated and/or processed with sulfur dioxide

- Farm-raised fish and meats . . . Animals that are not raised eating a diet that is natural to them get sick and pass on lots of inflammation-promoting Omega 6 fatty acids and microorganisms.

- Refined carbohydrates . . . These are your breads, flours, and baked goods and there is only one way for them to be digested and assimilated: by being broken down into glucose and fructose. Avoid them as much as possible, especially during the initial weight-loss phase. Get your fiber from massive amounts of vegetables and a little fruit.

- All cheap, processed foods . . . Potato chips, muffins, cookies, sugared yogurt, cereals . . . Ditch them all! That includes the "fat free" versions which are loaded with extra sugar and salt.

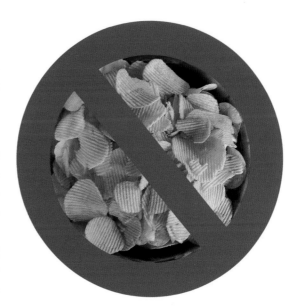

- Genetically Modified Organisms (GMOs) . . . Stay away from these when possible and opt for organic products. The testing standards for GMOs are poor, and they haven't been around long enough for us to know about the long-term effects on human beings. But, what we do know is somewhat frightening!

- Fast Food . . . Or, the "Anti-Nutrition!"

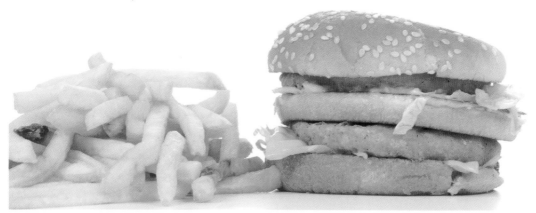

Luscious and Vitalizing

- Vegetables, vegetables, and more vegetables!

- Colorful fruits and berries that contain phytonutrients

- Wild salmon, halibut, mackerel, sardines, and other wild, deep sea fish

- Free-range, hormone-free, antibiotic-free, grass-fed meats

- Raw nuts and seeds, unsalted

- Legumes, unprocessed and in small amounts, as long as you do not have food sensitivities

Beginning this journey may seem overwhelming and very daunting. But, as you add amazing new foods to your diet that are luscious and satiating, you naturally will crowd out the old foods. You just will not have enough room in your diet for the health-destroying foods. Your taste will change quickly ... and I mean this literally. You no longer will need refined sugars to satisfy your "sweet tooth." Fruit will begin to taste incredibly sweet. You won't need as much salt to flavor foods. The natural, nutty flavors and spices will overwhelm your taste buds with joy. And remember . . . it is easier to replace a bad habit with a good one than it is to eliminate a bad habit. No one wants to feel that they are being deprived!

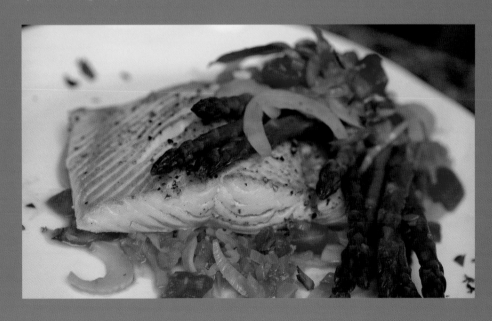

Breaking up Is NOT Hard to Do

Swap This for That

- Try green tea or herbal tea with a few drops of Stevia instead of coffee. My favorite "comfort drink" is sugar-free, steamed almond milk with a bag of green chai tea and a few drops of cinnamon-flavored Stevia. This is a guilt-free "tea latte." (My favorite brand of Stevia is Sweet Leaf.)

- Try using a little light coconut milk in your tea or coffee instead of half and half or soy creamer.

- Drink sparkling water sweetened with root beer-flavored Stevia instead of diet soda.

- Try sparkling water with a squeeze of lemon or lime and a few drops of lemon-flavored Stevia in place of wine. This is a great drink for parties when you want a "drink" to be social but you don't want to consume alcohol.

- Try almond milk instead of dairy milk and soy milk.

- Replace candy with "Brain On Joy" bars. These taste exactly like an "Almond Joy" candy bar, but they are sweetened with maltitol. This is a great alternative when you have PMS! But, they still should be eaten only as an occasional treat. These can be found on the website www. amenclinics.com.

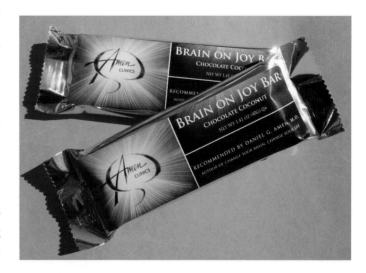

- Replace ice cream with "Avocado Gelato." (See Page 197 in the cookbook for this guilt-free dessert.)

- Eat ½ apple with almond butter instead of cookies and candy.

- Eat ¼ cup raw, unsalted nuts and one piece of 70 percent low-sugar dark chocolate instead of muffins, cookies, and candy.

- Try salsa or sugar-free catsup instead of the catsups and barbeque sauces that are filled with sugar and red dye. You also can look online for great sugar-free catsup recipes.

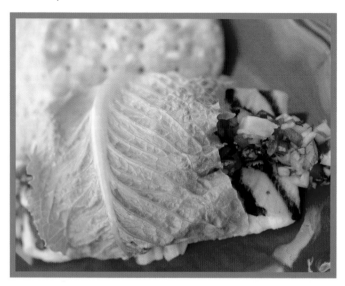

- Use Vegenaise, guacamole, or hummus instead of mayonnaise.

- Avocados, nuts, and seeds are great alternatives to cheese on your salads.

- Use lettuce instead of bread for sandwiches and wraps.

- Try Shirataki noodles instead of pasta.

A Note About Shirataki Noodles . . .

By far, one my best discoveries is using Shirataki noodles to replace pasta. Shirataki noodles are made from the root of the konnyaku imo plant (a yam-like vegetable). They are inexpensive and can be purchased in bulk online or at Whole Foods. These noodles are virtually calorie free and fat free, and they contain only 3 grams of carbs for an entire package! Also, the carbs they do contain are soluble fiber. This slows digestion and allows for slower absorption of sugar. My favorite brand is "Miracle Noodle."

They do have a slightly different consistency than regular pasta so I wouldn't suggest eating them plain. But, if you add a nutritious sauce, they are great! I knew I was on to something when my husband said, "This is the first time I have eaten noodles that I didn't feel hungry before I even finished my meal" (which happens when a heavy carb load interferes with the satiety signal that should go to your brain).

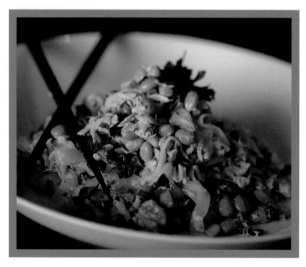

Prepare Your Life, Your Kitchen and Your Food for Success

"If you fail to plan, you plan to fail."- Unknown

Know Your Triggers and Come up With a Plan: Tana's Tricks for Thwarting Triggers

1. Going to the movies used to be a constant battle. The ADD in me just won't let me sit still without munching on something. It used to be candy and popcorn. Now I plan ahead by taking a few cherries, grapes (with seeds), or some other fruit, and a handful of nuts. Cut-up vegetables and a small container of split pea hummus are another great alternative. I also take herbal tea or lemon water with me.

2. Birthday cake! For me, birthday cake (or any cake) used to be like crack cocaine for a junkie! After kicking my addiction, I realized that I still needed a plan. If I am going to a party where there will be cake, I make sure that I have had protein and some good fat before arriving. This increases satiety and decreases cravings. I always take my own dessert as well. Usually, I take some raw nuts and seeds, fruit, or a "Brain On Joy" bar. If I am feeling a little weak for some reason (PMS), I leave the party right after they sing but before they serve the cake.

3. Disneyland is not the happiest place on earth when you are trying to eat well! Whenever I go there or to other amusement parks, I always bring my own snacks, as listed above.

4. Basically, I make sure to have healthy snacks with me wherever I go! I encourage you to come up with a list of snacks and always have them with you too.

Be Conscious and Thoughtful About Your Food Choices

Begin to think of yourself as **"A Living Example of Health and Fitness."** Take on an identity of health, vitality, and energy! People often ask me if I am a vegan or a "raw food" person. I avoid being tagged with those labels and I focus, instead, on being a healthy person.

For me, I make the healthiest choices that I can by utilizing the information and resources that I have at the time. I also know what feels right. At home, my diet tends to gravitate naturally toward raw, plant-based foods for probably about 70-80 percent of the foods that I eat. I just feel the most energy when I eat this way.

Be a leader in your own life, then you can lead your family, your friends, and your community.

As a person who struggled with an abusive relationship with food for years, I can't begin to tell you how good it feels to be free of the addictions and frustrations surrounding food. But, I do know that once you make the commitment to a healthier lifestyle, you occasionally may make a decision to eat something that isn't "the healthiest choice." This happens, but I urge you to take control by making it a conscious decision instead of an impulsive one. Then, if it does happen, do not begin the process of self-loathing because you didn't eat perfectly. This will get you nowhere!

Perfection is an excuse for people not to strive for success.

- *Perfection is unattainable.*

- *Pay attention to your internal dialogue.*

- *Kill the negative self-talk that does nothing to empower you.*

- *Your subconscious doesn't have a sense of humor. Sow thoughts according to the results you expect to reap.*

- *If you make a misstep, tell yourself you will make a healthier choice the next time . . . then drop it! Do not continue to focus on it.*

- *Focus on being a "Living Example of Health and Fitness."*

Having the mental tools—knowledge and good intentions—will not carry you far enough if you do not have the physical tools in place for truly changing your brain and getting thinner, smarter, and happier. As part of your quest for a life of health and vitality, you also must plan ahead and have your kitchen and your food plan organized and ready! The following is a brief outline for optimizing your success:

Your Kitchen . . .

1. *Throw out the unhealthy, processed foods that are taking up room in your pantry and make room for the wonderful new additions you will be purchasing.* This will enable you to make conscious decisions more easily without falling into the trap of impulsive, mindless snacking. Make one decision (not to have it in your house) instead of thirty decisions (to stay away from temptations that are in your pantry). Then, if you do make a decision to eat something not on your program, don't make it easy on yourself — make it so that you have to go out and get it. When you are done, get rid of it. Do not bring it back to your home!

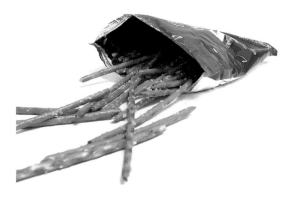

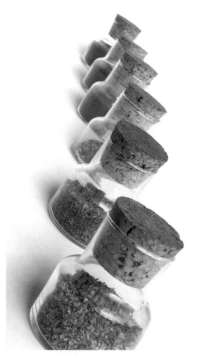

2. *Organize your spice cabinet with the list of brain healthy spices discussed in detail in "The Amen Solution."* We use a lot of these spices throughout the recipes. Though we prefer to cook with fresh herbs when possible, it is useful to have dried herbs and spices available for convenience and saving time. Here are some of our favorites for brain health:

   Saffron - Improves memory and helps support a positive mood.

   Curry - A potent antioxidant and anti-inflammatory agent that helps to decrease the plaques thought to be responsible for Alzheimer's disease.

   Oregano - A potent antioxidant that may help with PMS and insomnia.

Basil - A potent antioxidant that improves blood flow to the brain and may help memory.

Cinnamon - Improves working memory and the ability to pay attention.

Garlic - Improves blood flow to the brain and increases immunity.

Ginger - A potent anti-aging and anti-inflammatory agent.

Thyme - Increases DHA (an important fat) in the brain.

Sage - Improves memory and overall mental functioning.

Rosemary - An antioxidant and anti-inflammatory agent.

Marjoram - Promotes healthy digestion and can soothe minor digestive upsets.

Sea Salt - It must not have been bleached or chemically altered.

3. *Purchase plenty of travel-size storage containers and keep them in a handy location in your kitchen.* Immediately pack leftovers in the containers so you are ready to go the next day. This will ensure that you are prepared with a good supply of healthy options. You are less likely to find yourself so hungry that you are tempted to pull into the nearest fast food drive-thru.

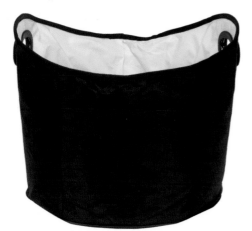

4. *Always have an ice chest out and ready to pack.* Have frozen ice packs ready to go. Take a small ice chest filled with healthy food whenever you leave the house.

5. *Stock your kitchen with healthy foods in "snack size packs" that are ready to grab and go.* I even travel long distances with enough veggies, hummus, fruit, raw nuts, and seeds (unsalted), etc. to last at least two or three days (until I can get to a grocery store).

Your Food . . .

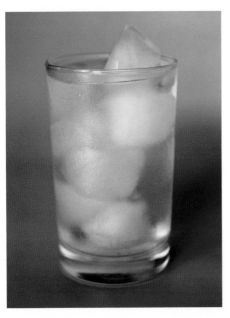

1. *Make sure you drink enough water.* Divide your body weight in half and convert it into ounces (If you weigh 160 pounds, you should drink 80 ounces of water). That's how many ounces of water you need to drink in a day. Also, be conscious of electrolyte replacement, especially if you are an athlete or a very active person. There are waters available that have electrolytes in them and no sugar. Avoid commercial electrolyte drinks that have added sugars and high fructose corn syrup.

Other beverages don't count toward your daily water consumption. Coffee, tea, and caffeinated soda don't count. They are diuretics and actually act to dehydrate you. You need to drink water!

You may add a little lemon to your water. My husband doesn't like to drink water, but if I add fresh lemon juice and a few drops of lemon flavored Stevia he will drink it down like lemonade!

2. *Add greens to your water or smoothie at least one time each day.* Freeze-dried greens can be found at any health food store. One of my favorite brands is "Green Vibrance."

Since most people do not get close to the minimum recommended servings of fruits and vegetables (which is a low recommendation for optimal health), adding greens to your water is a fabulous way to give your energy a quick boost. This also gives your body a nice shot of up to 25 billion probiotics and too many varieties of plant extracts to mention. While this is not a replacement for fresh vegetables and fruits, it is an awesome supplement. It also gives you a much needed fiber boost.

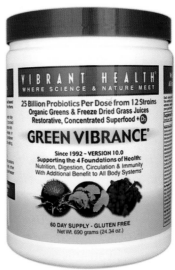

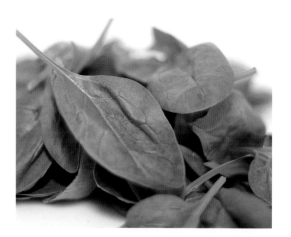

3. **Purchase fresh, organic produce when possible.** The pesticide residual from non-organic produce is more concentrated in some fruits and vegetables than others and can lead to many brain and health issues. When you can't choose fresh produce, try to use organic, frozen fruits and vegetables. Do not use canned fruits and vegetables.

4. **Don't cook any foods at high temperatures using olive oil or any oil that has a low smoking point.** Choose oils that have a high smoking temperature such as coconut oil, grape seed oil, organic butter or ghee. To eliminate confusion, I usually just use coconut oil. However, we try to limit the amount of oil we use in cooking altogether so we opt for sautéing in vegetable broth as much as possible.

It is important to get enough essential fatty acids in your diet, though. Healthy oils are a great way to do that, so we add enough oil to foods that are not cooked, or after cooking. This way it isn't necessary for us to get our daily essential fatty acids from cooked oils that actually may be doing more harm than good.

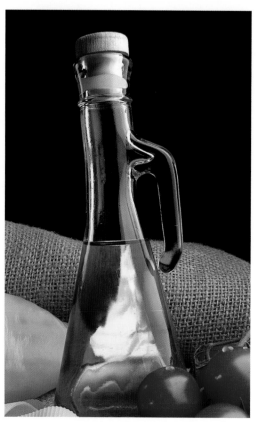

5. **Limit the amount of fattening, sugar-loaded condiments you use.** Try swapping avocado, hummus, or Earth Balance® (in limited amounts) for butter. Stevia is a healthy alternative to sugar. Vegannaise is a good substitute for mayonnaise, but it is still fattening and processed, so use it sparingly. I usually use salsa in place of catsup in order to eliminate the sugar. For a comprehensive list of alternatives, see the chart "Swap This for That" on page 48.

6. *Be careful about using pre-cut and pre-packed onions, garlic, ginger, and other herbs that are processed and preserved in chemicals that are often harmful, or at least, not helpful.* Use fresh products as often as possible.

7. *When you prepare foods, make certain that you prepare enough so that you definitely will have leftovers.*

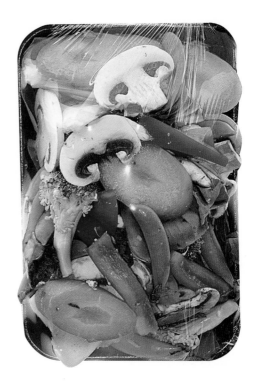

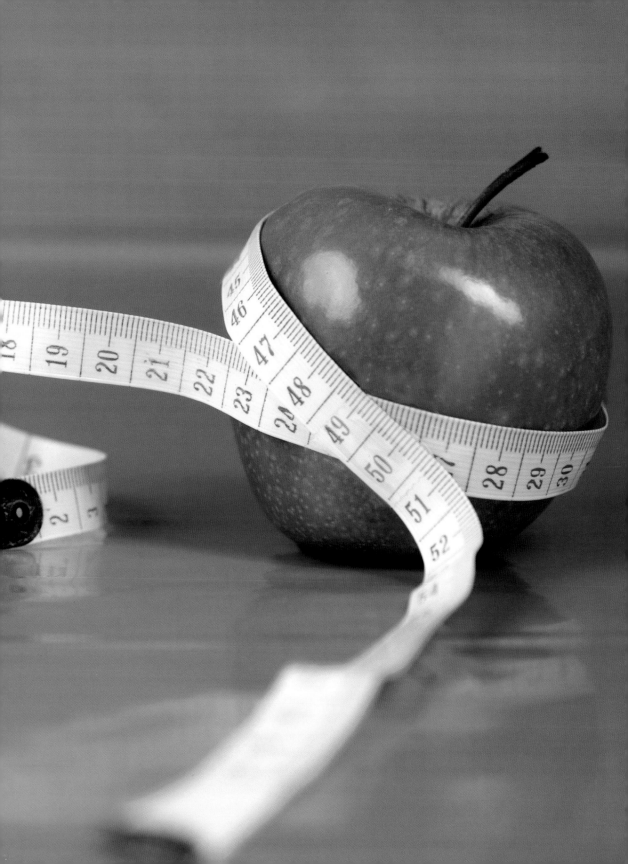

Chapter 4

NOW THAT I KNOW WHAT TO EAT, HOW SHOULD I EAT? Basic Facts, Tips for Success & What Vegetarians Should Know

Chapter 4

NOW THAT I KNOW WHAT TO EAT, HOW SHOULD I EAT? Basic Facts, Tips for Success & What Vegetarians Should Know

Eat Like a Gorilla

If you want to know how to eat, the plain and simple truth is that you should eat like a gorilla! Right about now, you might be saying "WHAT?" but, trust me, this is not as crazy as it sounds. We share a nearly identical DNA and digestive system structure with gorillas. Since gorillas are the strongest mammals pound for pound—they have the ability to lift 10 times their body weight—we would do well to take a lesson from them in the strength department.

Gorillas eat less than 5 percent animal protein, but it turns out that this small amount of animal protein is vital to their health. They obtain this animal protein

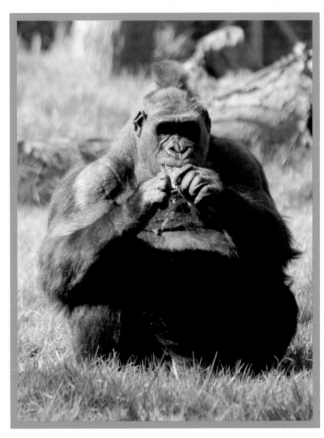

mostly in the form of the termites, small bugs, and worms that are on the plants they eat and from preening one another. Yet, it would be inaccurate to say that they are deficient in protein. On the contrary, gorillas get an amazing amount of plant-based protein. Many green leaves are up to 50 percent protein and are loaded with micronutrients. These powerful beasts eat up to 16 pounds of leaves and berries every day, and they manage to include nearly 200 different varieties of plants in their diets! This rounds out their diet nicely.

While we don't have the time or the energy to sit around eating greens all day, and therefore most of us will opt to eat a little more animal protein than gorillas because our digestive tracts are smaller and can't accommodate 16 pounds of greens, we can take a lesson from our "shoulder joint" sharing friends (a unique feature that gives gorillas the ability to pull leaves from trees). We need to increase the amount of greens we eat . . . dramatically!

Some experts do argue with this because gorillas differ from people in that they are built for strength while human beings are built for endurance. These experts point to the fact that one of the differences between gorilla DNA and human DNA is that we have more copies of the gene for digesting starch. This, of course, leads us to believe that we can eat more starch than a gorilla. The question then becomes, Should we eat more starch than gorillas?

To answer that question, I want to remind you of the correlation between food production methods and the rise of disease over the course of human history. It wasn't until the advent of farming around five thousand years ago that grains came on the scene in a big way. But, farming was really hard work! Farmers and peasants burned off what they ate—when they even had enough to eat. Yet, along with farming of grains (and other crops), we also have our first records of heart disease, diabetes, cancer, and obesity – and this was when the grains were wholesome, un-refined, and not mass produced! We also know, though, that the people who were overweight and dying of these diseases (for the most part) were the aristocracy and the wealthy! With the advent of farming, the people who didn't have to work for their dinner paid for it in a whole new way... with chronic illness!

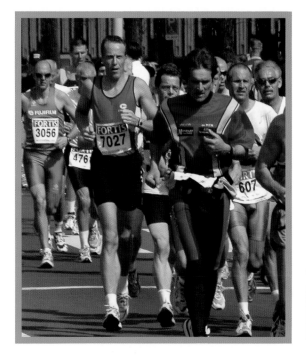

So, if you perform intense manual labor or you are a marathon runner, by all means, feel free to increase your whole grains and wholesome starchy carbs a little bit. The rest of you should cut way back on grains and starchy carbs and take a lesson from our furry friends. Strength training is one of the healthiest forms of training for longevity, and the diet that best supports this is a diet that is similar to a gorilla's... a whole lot of greens, nuts, seeds, fruit, and some animal protein.

One way to accomplish this is through "green smoothies," green juices, and daily shots of wheat grass. I also want you to know that spinach and broccoli have more protein than most cuts of meats, pound for pound. Of course, it takes a massive amount of spinach to make a pound. But that's the point! Like the gorillas, you should be filling up on "free" calories that are jam-packed with micronutrients.

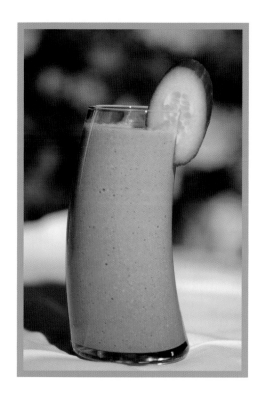

In the *Eat healthy With the Brain Doctor's Wife Cookbook* designed to accompany this coaching guide, you will notice that nearly every meal is an intentional balance of protein, fat, fiber, and high-quality carbohydrates. We suggest that about 70 percent of your daily food consumption comes from live, water-rich sources of food. This means vegetables, vegetable juice, a little fruit, nuts, seeds (especially sprouted) . . . and more vegetables!

The remaining 30 percent of your daily food intake should come from "concentrated" foods, which are foods that are cooked and do not have a high water content, live

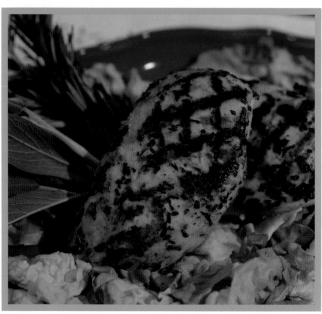

enzymes, or phytonutrients. The foods in this category are animal protein, soy protein, grains, and legumes. In creating and balancing meals in this way, you manage the Glycemic Load (GL) of your food intake. When you follow this formula, you design meals and snacks that are balanced for optimal brain function and, consequently, physical function. What's good for your brain is good for your body!

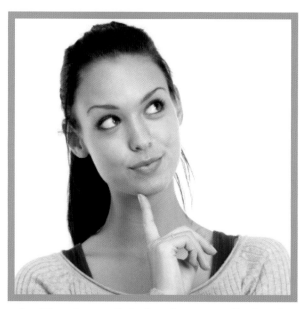

What Are the Facts About a "Healthy Lifestyle" and Why Is This so Confusing?

With the constant barrage of conflicting messages about health and fitness flooding our televisions and bookstores, it's no wonder that so many people are confused about what is fact and what is fiction when it comes to health. Truthfully, one of the sources of this confusion is that there is not one perfect solution that fits every person. **One diet does not fit all—and that is why *The Amen Solution* is not a diet!** Gluten and grains will literally make some people act crazy and feel very sick so they must eat more meat, vegetables, and fruit. Other people thrive on a vegetarian diet and feel awful when they eat any meat.

This means that it is essential for you to know yourself better if you truly want to improve your health, your vitality, and your relationship with food. As the first step in this journey, make it a point to discover if you have hidden food allergies or delayed reaction food sensitivities. Otherwise, your efforts to improve your health will be totally sabotaged if you eat foods that negatively affect your body.

Meet Kim . . .

Kim is a perfect example of the need to know your own body better. I met Kim when she was 38 years old. She was a great athlete and very fit. But I noticed that she had pretty bad acne and a lot of facial hair. She also complained about her irregular periods and terrible mood swings. Kim wanted to know if I thought that my husband could help her, and if I knew of any doctors that could help her with her hormones. She also asked me for advice about changing her diet.

When Kim came to me with all of this, she felt like she was falling apart on the inside even though she looked very fit on the outside. This was all the more perplexing to her because she believed that she was eating a very healthy diet. She was a vegan who ate lots of fruits and vegetables, pasta, soy, whole grain breads, legumes, and rice. However, she also admitted that she had an insatiable sweet tooth and a craving for caffeine all the time. As a result, she was experiencing major dips in her energy and she suffered from "mental fog."

I suggested that she see a hormone specialist that I know and be tested for Polycystic Ovarian Syndrome (PCOS). The acne, facial hair, and lack of periods were a dead giveaway that she was experiencing a problem with her hormones. She also had a soft abdomen in spite of the fact that she trained very hard with weights and that the rest of her body was really toned. This is often a sign of elevated levels of cortisol.

As I suspected, Kim's evaluation with the hormone specialist revealed that she indeed had PCOS. This was bad news. The external symptoms of PCOS are unpleasant, but the internal symptoms are dangerous. Kim had high cholesterol, high triglycerides, and insulin resistance. So, in spite of being thin and eating a fairly "healthy" diet, Kim was a step away from being diabetic!

I also wanted Kim to have a full physical. She had an evaluation at the Amen Clinics. A brain scan revealed decreased activity in Kim's frontal lobes. Her blood work revealed very low vitamin D levels. Her food sensitivity test revealed sensitivities to gluten, dairy, soy, and many legumes. Also, it seemed likely that Kim was suffering from "leaky gut." Nothing like letting it all hang out! Her profile looked eerily like my own and like the profiles of the many women we see who complain of irritability, lack of focus, lack of energy, mental fog, and a host of physical ailments.

Kim needed help! We suggested a brain healthy program for Kim and the hormone specialist gave her some suggestions as well. In addition, my husband suggested that I give her some coaching about how her food sensitivities were affecting her health and how she could adopt a new lifestyle.

Within one week Kim called me because she was excited that she had lost her "sweet tooth!" She also told me that her mental fog had disappeared and that her energy level had improved dramatically and was holding steady! She no longer was experiencing dips throughout the day. Then, within two months, her periods were normal, her triglycerides were under 100, and she was sleeping much better.

Now, six months later, Kim has successfully reduced the amount of Metformin that she was prescribed for the blood sugar problems associated with her PCOS . . . And she is confident that she will be able to eliminate this medication altogether if she continues to follow her new lifestyle. Also, although she didn't need to lose weight, Kim has gained lean muscle mass by changing her diet. She has lost that "soft" look around the abdomen. Her skin is clear and smooth. Better yet, Kim says that she has never felt better and she looks vibrant and healthy!

Kim's story is personal to me because it is so similar to my own. It also serves as a great example to all of us about how our individual chemistry goes a long way in determining how we should eat. However, I also want you to know that when your remove the hype, headlines, and hoopla from the barrage of diet advice that bombards you every day, there are core truths about diet and nutrition that can apply to every person. It's just not that easy to get this unbiased information unless you are actively searching, but it does exist!

These are the principles at the core of The Amen Solution. It doesn't really matter whether you are a vegan, a vegetarian, or a meat-eating cave man, it is very clear that processed foods, cheap oils, and a diet that is high in sugar and omega-6 fatty acids will make you fat and lead to chronic illness. It is also clear that, no matter who you are, whole, live, water-rich foods that are filled with phytonutrients, vitamins, and minerals will give you energy, make you lean, and help you to thrive mentally, physically, and emotionally.

So, for all of the confusing information about nutrition and lifestyle plans, there is a solid base of factual information that you can use to guide your quest for health and overall wellness.

Have You Ever Seen a "Sweet Tooth?"

I began wondering where the expression "sweet tooth" originated from, and more important, why some people seem to struggle with one for a lifetime, while other people are not much concerned with sugar at all. Once again, my research lead me back to nutrition, or actually to "anti-nutrition." As you can see, limiting carbs is a commonality amongst most the leading diet plans. You may recall from earlier in this book that once you have eaten more carbohydrates than your liver can store (in the form of gly-

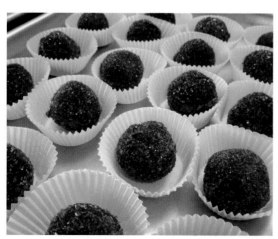

cogen), the excess carbs are converted to palmitic acid (PA). This PA thwarts the satiety signal to the brain because it makes us less sensitive to the satiety hormone leptin.

Under normal circumstances, your body is designed to tell you that you are full if your blood sugar is high. But, if you eat an excessive amount of carbohydrates and your liver and other cells have nowhere to store them, they will be converted to PA and you will feel hungry in spite of the fact that you have just eaten and your blood sugar is high. Even worse, you will be hungry for more carbohydrates because your insulin is also elevated and this has signaled to your body that your blood sugar is low. You end up with a "sweet tooth" as a result. This is the same phenomenon that causes Type 2 Diabetes! *So . . . Find your "sweet tooth" and pull the darn thing out!*

Common Characteristics of Leading Nutritional Programs...

- Eliminate sugar from your diet as much possible.

- Avoid processed foods (especially carbs and cheap oils) as much as possible.

- Eliminate refined and starchy carbs as much as possible.

- Get the bulk of your carbs from vegetables and fruits.

- When choosing complex carbs, choose whole or sprouted grains (such as barley, brown rice, and quinoa) and eat them in small amounts.

- Avoid products containing gluten when possible. Most people have some level of sensitivity to gluten. Get checked if you suspect any sensitivity.

- Eat small meals frequently throughout the day.

- Get the proper amount of protein (not too much and certainly not too little) with each meal. This can be done whether you are a vegan or a meat lover.

- Have your relevant medical numbers checked: blood pressure, heart rate, triglycerides, cholesterol, Hg A1C, vitamin D, thyroid levels, etc.

- Consume enough essential fatty acids, especially omega-3 fatty acids.

- Take proper supplements for your individual needs: Everyone should take fish oil (or a good source of omega-3 fatty acids), vitamin D, and a multiple vitamin.

- Have an informed coach who can help you sift through the diet information garbage in order for you to find the pearls.

- Have a mentor or a buddy who can help you stay on track.

Tips for Success:
How to Eat and How to Prepare Your Foods in Ways that Optimize Brain Function and Weight Loss

1. **Do not skip breakfast! This truly is your most important meal of the day.** Smoothies made with raw fruit, veggies, nuts, and protein are my favorite meal for starting the day.

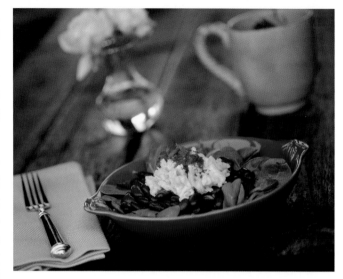

2. **Eliminate bread completely for the first 30 days if possible.** (The first two weeks are the most critical.) Use iceberg or Romaine lettuce for sandwiches and wraps. If you must eat bread occasionally, opt for gluten-free or flourless bread such as Ezekiel bread, and make it a rare treat.

3. **Minimize coffee consumption.** Believe me, this one is personal for me! There is a lot of controversy over whether or not coffee is a problem, and I have sought out every known reason for making coffee drinking all right. But the

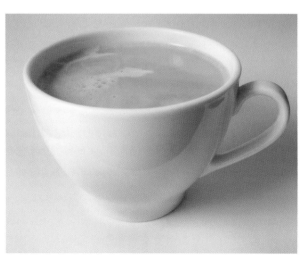

fact remains that, although coffee does contain some antioxidants, it is also highly acidic. This is not good for your system. Also, coffee is not good for your brain. That caffeine "jolt" momentarily may wake you up, but it quickly acts a vasoconstrictor and decreases blood flow to the brain. Within a short time, you need another cup of Joe to wake you up again. Finally, if you use dairy creamers or milk in your coffee, the dairy binds to the antioxidants that the coffee does contain and changes their properties completely. So, if you still feel that you must have your coffee, try switching to almond or coconut milk. And if you drink coffee as a comfort "food," try drinking "half caf" (half caffeinated and half decaffeinated) as an alternative.

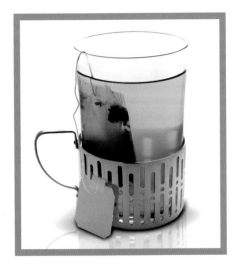

4. **Drink green tea!** Though green tea has a little caffeine, it's about one-third of the caffeine in coffee and the tea is full of antioxidant properties. For those of you trying to break up with coffee this is good news. Also, studies have shown that people who drink three cups of green tea every day have younger-looking DNA. And green tea comes in lots of great flavors but, just like with coffee, ditch the dairy creamers and replace them with almond or coconut milk.

5. **Do not allow yourself to get hungry.** Eat *small* amounts at least every three hours. This might be our greatest challenge because we have been programmed to eat until we feel completely full. Instead, we need to retrain our bodies to eat just enough. Remember, you are going to eat again shortly! Eating this way will keep your blood sugar stable and your hormones balanced.

6. **Eat small amounts of lean protein throughout the day.** When you are in the initial phase of your weight-loss program, eating more protein and less carbs will actually speed up your weight loss. That's why high-protein diets always work . . . at first! However, there is a long-term price to pay. The energy that is needed by your body to digest all the extra protein (especially large amounts of animal protein) generates a lot of heat and is believed to speed up the aging process. So, once your goal is reached, you should continue to eat protein throughout the day, but you should also consider reducing the amount of that protein. Satisfy your hunger by increasing your consumption of live foods instead.

In his book, **Dr. Gundry's Diet Evolution,** *Dr. Steven Gundry, an expert in genetic evolution, restorative health and longevity, explains the importance of reducing the amount of animal protein we consume once we have reached our optimal weight.*

7. **Do not deep fry foods.** This diminishes nearly all of the nutritional value of your food and it adds excessive amounts of unhealthy fat (usually trans fat) to your diet. It also can have serious consequences for brain function, heart health, and the size of your waistline. As we covered in Chapter 2, cooking oils pose serious threats to your health.

8. **Try to get a large portion of your veggies either raw or only lightly cooked (crunchy) most of the time.** Fried zucchini and onion rings do not figure into your daily servings of vegetables!

9. **When cooking vegetables, try lightly sautéing them in low-sodium vegetable broth instead of oil.** When using oil, limit it as much as possible. Most of us use far more oil than we need.

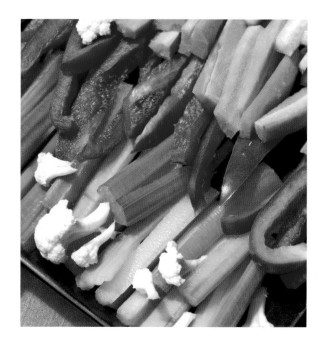

10. **There are some veggies, grains, and legumes that contain high concentrations of lectins, so these foods are much better for you when they are properly cooked.** Tomatoes, eggplant, and legumes are some examples.

11. **Eat fruit raw!** Chocolate covered strawberries don't count in your daily servings of fruit. Dried fruit, at best, is a highly concentrated sugar with the valuable water content removed, and, at worst, is harmful if it contains sulfur dioxide. It is sure to increase your triglycerides and your waistline!

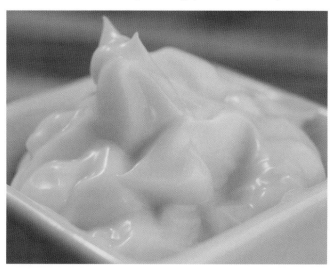

12. **Do not let your condiments sabotage your weight loss and your health.** Most people have no idea what is in their condiments. Take a look at the ingredients on your condiments and you will be surprised! Refer to the chart "Breaking up Is not Hard to Do" on page 63 for some alternative suggestions.

13. **Minimize alcohol consumption.** Contrary to what you hear, alcohol is not a health food! Even if it's true that it has some benefits for your heart, it definitely does not have benefits for your brain. There is no question that alcohol kills brain cells. It also impairs judgment and decreases inhibitions. One drink too many can have you making a decision that will ruin all your hard work! And since it is sugar, it makes you want more sugar. So, if you want wine, limit it to just a couple of glasses per week. In addition, many alcohols are made from grains so if you are gluten or lectin intolerant, alcohol can wreak havoc on your weight-loss plan and your health. If you must have a cocktail, drink tequila made from agave instead.

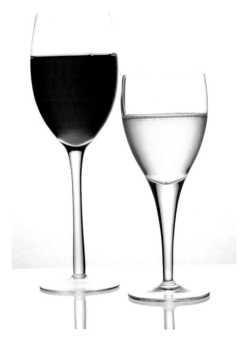

14. **Add freeze-dried greens and lemon to your water.** I know that I have mentioned this already, but I just cannot say enough about how important it is to stay hydrated! By adding lemon to your water at least once per day, you also can counter all the acid-forming foods we eat that make us sick and age our bodies... and it's refreshing! And by adding greens to your water at least once per day, you can chip away at the deficit in the amount of antioxidants, vitamins, and minerals that most of us have from not eating enough fruits and vegetables. My favorite brand of greens is "Green Vibrance" because it also contains probiotics. Be sure to read the ingredient list. It has LOTS of fruits and vegetable extracts so you must be sure that you are not allergic to any of the components. Also, if you really don't like the greens in your water, try adding them to smoothies instead.

Above all, the greatest tip for success is to focus on making health and nutrition a lifelong lifestyle and an exciting journey instead of a diet! Your beliefs about food and your state of mind have a powerful effect on how your body processes your food!

A Note for Vegetarians . . .

While vegans and vegetarians can find vibrant health, there is some evidence that following strict vegan or vegetarian diets can be problematic if you are not well informed and if you are not proactive with your nutritional program. Since non-meat eaters tend to supplement their diets with excessive amounts of soy, grains, pasta, and bread, they can end up with systemic inflammation, "mental fog," and muscle wasting. This also can lead to high cholesterol or high triglycerides in spite of the fact that many vegans and vegetarians don't eat many processed foods and are not overweight.

Also, while vegans and vegetarians can be thin, they often have roundness or flabbiness around their middles. This is from the elevated cortisol that is released when the system is flooded with too much sugar from the carbohydrates (rice, pasta, etc.) in their diets.

The vegans and vegetarians who tend to be the healthiest are those who eat a more "raw" diet of vegetable juices, nuts, seeds, raw or lightly cooked vegetables, a little fruit, and some whole grains (especially sprouted) while only supplementing with soy. Although the total caloric intake of nuts, seeds, and avocados is higher than grains and bread, you will lose weight faster eating this way because you will decrease inflammation, reduce blood insulin levels (hence insulin resistance), and decrease cortisol. Also, grains, breads, and refined carbs will increase your appetite, while nuts, seeds, and avocados will increase your satiety.

Most vegans and vegetarians know that their obvious challenge is protein. However, they also need to know that one of their greatest challenges is the imbalance in the omega-3 to omega-6 fatty acid ratio in their diet. This imbalance causes systemic inflammation. Omega-3 fatty acids are essential! For vegans and vegetarians who are willing to take a fish oil supplement, a lot of this systemic inflammation can be counteracted. Those who are not willing to take fish oil supplements can supplement with flax oil, or some of the other oil blends available, but they are inferior when it comes to the quality of omega-3 fatty acids. The following chart provides some additional tips for avoiding the omega-3/omega-6 fatty acid imbalance as well.

TIPS FOR VEGETARIANS AND VEGANS

1. **Eat small amounts of protein throughout the day by supplementing with vegetarian sources of protein powders and bars.** Watch the sugar! Olympian Labs makes a great pea protein. Applied Pro Sciences, endorsed by Tony Gonzalez, also makes a high-quality product. These are sweetened with Stevia. You can find them both online.

2. **Add more nuts, seeds, and avocados to your diet.** Chia seeds are 22 percent protein. Flax seeds are very high in omega-3 fatty acids.

3. **Eat eggs fortified with omega-3 fatty acids (from free-range, antibiotic-free chickens).**

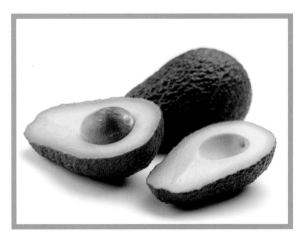

4. **If you are vegan, supplement with tofu or tempeh.** Avoid seitan since it is pure gluten. If you are unwilling to supplement with fish oil, find oil that is high in omega-3 and low in omega-6 fatty acids. Chances are good that you are already getting enough omega-6 fatty acids.

5. **Decrease the amount of bread, pasta, and refined grains you consume.**

6. **Increase the amount of greens you consume dramatically.** They are a great source of protein.

7. **Add wheat grass to your daily diet, twice a day if possible!** Start with 1 ounce and work up to 2 or 3 ounces. Green vegetable juices also are great!

8. **Get tested so that you will know your important lab values.** You can find these numbers in Appendix 2.

9. **Drink smoothies twice a day if you are having trouble eating a well-rounded diet.** They are a great way to add a protein supplement, greens, and other superfoods to your diet. But, don't add more than one piece of fruit.

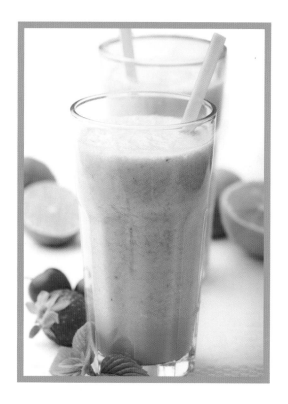

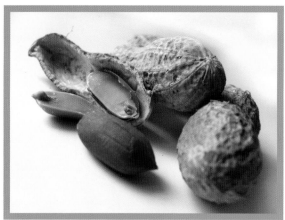

10. **Discover hidden food allergies and sensitivities with an IgG test.** Know if you are sensitive to gluten, wheat, yeast, legumes, dairy, and eggs. These do not always show up on traditional food allergy tests.

11. **Take the necessary supplements to keep you on track.**

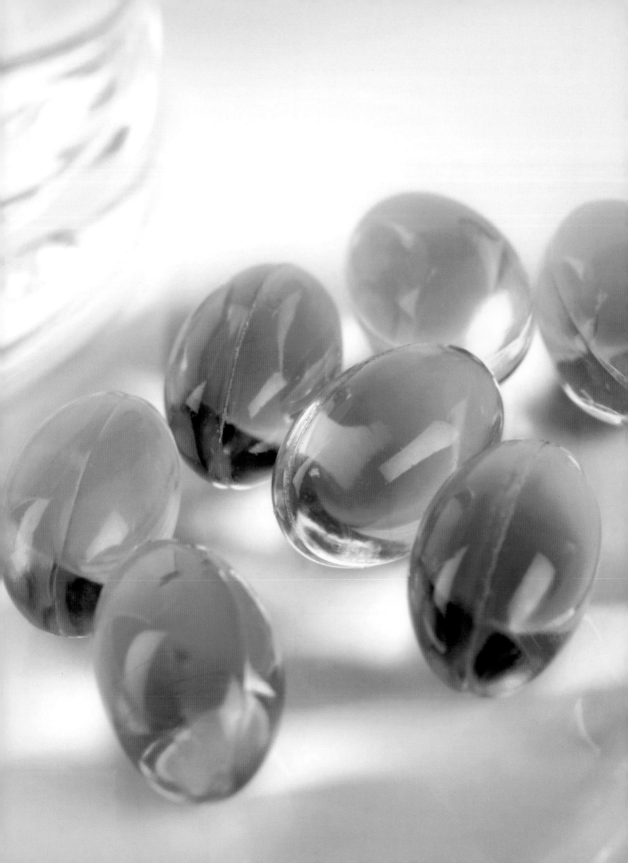

Chapter 5
SUPPLEMENTS:
A Cornerstone Of Success

Chapter 5

SUPPLEMENTS: A Cornerstone of Success

Even if you eat a perfect diet of 10 servings of organic fruits and vegetables every day, you eat the proper amounts of lean protein, you avoid sugar and other poisons, you drink 10 glasses of water every day, you sleep eight hours every night, and you have no stress (wow, I'm stressed just thinking about how far off the mark I am!), the fact remains that you live in a toxic world. We all are surrounded by air pollution, pesticides, and the innumerable other variables that constitute our daily lives. So, in reality, it is virtually impossible to receive all of the nutrients you need every day from your diet unless you live in the Garden of Eden!

Still, you may not be certain as to whether or not you want to take supplements (nutraceuticals) in order to bridge this gap. After all, we hear two myths about supplements:

1. *Supplements do nothing for you, so don't bother with them.*

2. *Supplements can't hurt you, so there's no harm in trying them.*

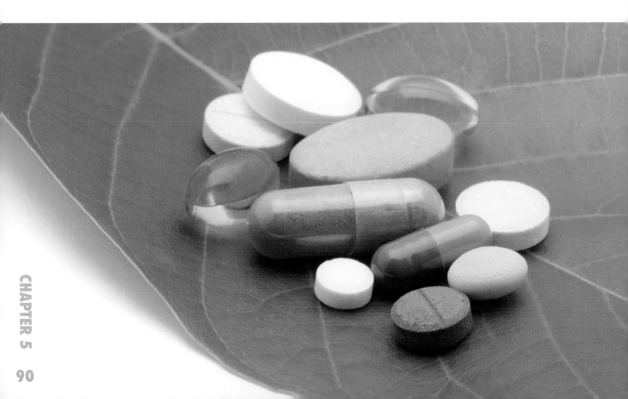

I cannot tell you that you should or should not make supplements a part of your daily diet, but I can tell you two truths about them:

1. *Most nutraceuticals definitely do something, so any choice that you make must be an informed decision! Get your information from an expert.*

2. *You can think of supplements as one "layer" in an overall healthy living program.*

When you start your quest for a life of health and well-being, you can take your program to whatever level you choose. Some of you will be ready to jump the canyon from the first day you embark on your healthy living journey. Others of you will engage in a longer process where you slowly incorporate new "layers" of healthy living choices over time. Regardless of how you choose to proceed, anything you do to improve

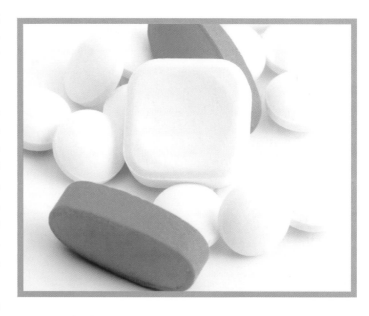

your health that you were not previously doing is a step in the right direction! If you do nothing more than stop the poisoning by cutting out processed foods, alcohol, and refined sugar, you will feel dramatically better and get results.

But, when you are ready to add a layer of healing by adding what's missing, you will find that most people benefit from some level of nutritional supplementation. Some of you have taken quite a bit of abuse over the years! It's different for everyone.

That said, I also believe that there a gazillion nutraceuticals on the market that you don't need for your basic health. I have nothing against them, per se. So, if you have a specific need or a belief in a certain supplement, go for it . . . as long as you know what you are doing. Don't ask the 17-year-old clerk at the store! It's a good idea to get your information about nutraceuticals from someone who has some knowledge about your individual brain type and metabolic needs instead.

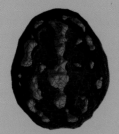 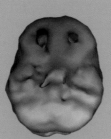 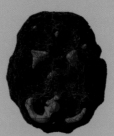 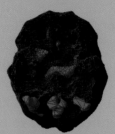
Nearly everyone should be on a basic supplement program that boosts their general nutrition and helps to alleviate the inflammation that plagues our systems. For these purposes, everyone should consider taking a good multi-vitamin, extra vitamin D, and fish oil.

- **Multi-vitamins:** These are fairly self-explanatory. Just make sure that you get a high-quality brand.

- **Vitamin D:** Most Americans have significantly low levels of vitamin D, either from spending too much time indoors or from wearing sunscreen. Vitamin D deficiency is associated with insulin resistance, diabetes, autoimmune disorders, depression, obesity, and infertility. A conservative dose is about 2,000 IU/day. A more average dose is about 5,000 IU/day. You must find out your current level of vitamin D in order to know how much of the supplement that you should take. Then, you should have your levels checked periodically. Also, if you require higher doses as a result of an autoimmune disorder or a severe deficiency, it's a good idea to consult with your physician. Vitamin D is a fat soluble vitamin.

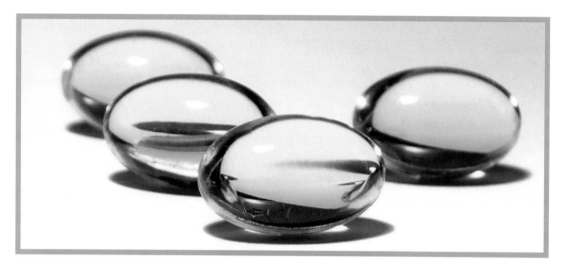

- **Fish oil:** This supplement is your best source for omega-3 fatty acids (EPA and DHA). Omega-3 fatty acid deficiency is associated with systemic inflammation, autoimmune disorders, increased risk of cancer, and neurodegeneration. It is not uncommon for people with chronic disease, systemic inflammation and obesity to supplement with up to 15g-20g/day of fish oil for the first month or so until their inflammation decreases. For healthy people, doses can vary from 3g-6g/day depending upon a person's size, lifestyle, and physical condition. Be sure to get a high-quality, ultra-refined fish oil to avoid the toxins, mercury, and digestive issues that can be associated with cheaper brands.

Beyond this basic plan for supplementation, you may want to investigate and consider the following supplements:

Alpha-lipoic acid: Made naturally in the body, alpha-lipoic acid may protect against cell damage in a variety of conditions. There is strong evidence that alpha-lipoic acid supports stable blood sugar levels, which helps to decrease cravings and tendencies to overeat. Studies have shown that it improves insulin sensitivity and may be effective in treating type 2 diabetes. The typical recommended adult dose is 100 mg twice a day.

Chromium: Supplementation with chromium picolinate has been shown to effectively modulate carbohydrate cravings and appetite, which is beneficial to managing both diabetes and depression. The typical recommended adult dosage is 200 to 600 micrograms a day.

DL-phenylalanine: This is an essential amino acid (cannot be produced by the body) and thus must be obtained through the diet. There is evidence that phenylalanine can increase mental alertness, release hormones affecting appetite, and reduce drug and alcohol cravings. There have been reports that L-phenylalanine can promote high blood pressure in those predisposed to hypertension. Persons who have PKU (phenylketonuria) cannot use phenylalanine. This includes those born with a genetic deficiency that prevents them from metabolizing phenylalanine. The typical recommended starting dosage for adults is 500 mg a day, and slowly work up to 1,500 mg a day.

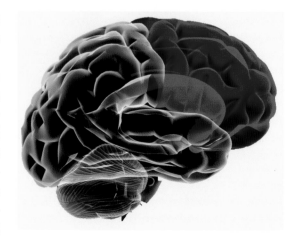

N-acetyl-cysteine (NAC): NAC is an amino acid that is needed to produce glutathione, a very powerful antioxidant. Recently, NAC has been studied as a treatment for drug addiction, as it functions to restore levels of the excitatory neurotransmitter glutamate in the reward center of the brain. A growing body of research has found that NAC can reduce cravings for cocaine, heroin, and cigarettes and decrease the risk for relapse. Considering that some foods activate the same areas of the brain as cocaine, it may be that NAC can also be helpful in reducing food cravings. Other research concludes that NAC shows promise for the treatment of compulsive behavior problems. The typical adult dose is 600 to 1,200 mg twice a day to curb cravings.

B Vitamins: The B vitamins play an integral role in the functioning of the nervous system and help the brain synthesize neurotransmitters that affect mood and thinking. Some research indicates that supplementation with some of the B vitamins may fight depression. The typical adult dose of B6 is 25 to 50 mg. For B12, it is 250 mcg.

Magnesium: Magnesium is a mineral that is essential to good health as it is needed for more than three hundred biochemical reactions in the body. It has been shown to be helpful in calming anxiety and balancing the brain's pleasure centers, which can help reduce cravings. The typical adult dose is 400-1,000 mg daily, divided into three doses. It is best to take with calcium as these minerals work synergistically. Magnesium is usually half of your total calcium intake.

Melatonin: Melatonin is a hormone made in the brain that helps regulate other hormones and maintains the body's sleep cycle. Darkness stimulates the production of melatonin while light decreases its activity. Melatonin is a strong antioxidant, and there is some evidence that it may help strengthen the immune system. It has also been shown to have powerful neuroprotective effects both as an antioxidant and in the prevention of plaque formation as observed in Alzheimer's disease. The best approach for dosing melatonin is to begin with very low doses. Start with 1 mg an

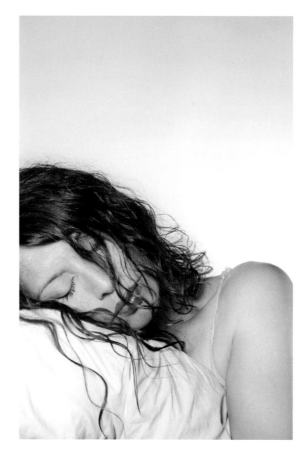

hour before bedtime. You can increase it to 6 mg for adults.

For more detailed information about supplements, read **The Amen Solution.**

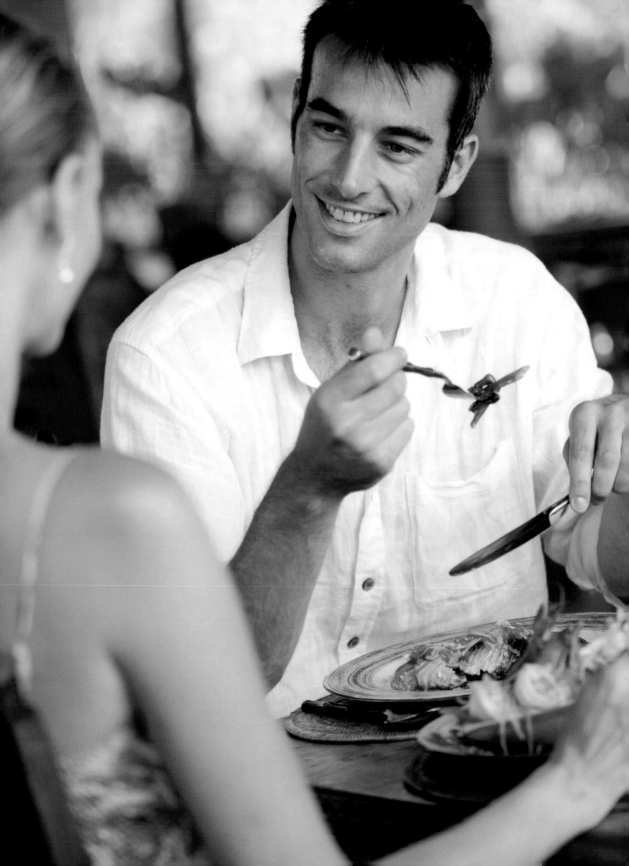

Chapter 6

OUT AND ABOUT:

How to Succeed in a World That Is Trying to Sabotage You

Chapter 6

OUT AND ABOUT: How to Succeed in a World That Is Trying to Sabotage You

While the way we eat in the Amen household may not be mainstream, it does seem to be slowly catching on. For a long time, though, I found it difficult to eat out at restaurants without feeling stress. I knew that they would have things on the menu that I did not want to put in my body, and I knew that they would not have things on the menu that I did want to put in my body. Hidden sugar, salt, and fat are everywhere these days! I wasn't willing to blow all my hard work for

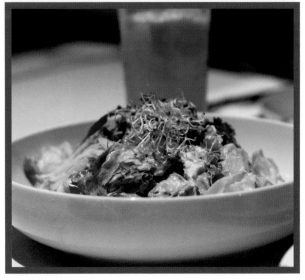

one night of dining out so, eventually, we just began to eat out less and less.

However, we really did not want to give up on the social aspect of the dining out experience, so I went on a mission to solve this dilemma. If you are changing your lifestyle for the first time and you are beginning to lose weight, then you understand how truly difficult it is to eat properly once you are outside of your own kitchen.

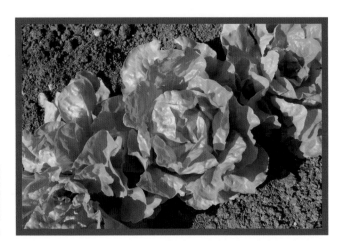

Both our society and the food companies who feed us are all too happy to sabotage our attempts to get healthy. As a result, you must be proactive and take your health into your own hands. Here are a few tips for being out and about that work for me . . .

1. *Plan ahead by finding three restaurants in your area that serve organic, locally grown produce; hormone-free, antibiotic-free, grass-fed meats; and wild fish.* Maybe you even can find a restaurant that serves an amazing "raw cuisine."

2. *Be proactive and choose the restaurant when you are eating out with friends.* If you let others make restaurant choices, you will be caught off guard.

3. *Make the healthiest choice possible when you are not in an ideal situation by ordering a big salad with olive oil and lemon or with the dressing on the side.* Steamed veggies and baked potatoes (go easy on potatoes) are fairly

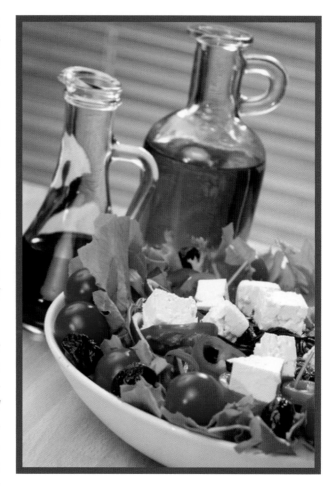

universal. And check out the appetizers, the "Small Bites," and the side order menus. You often will find things like brown rice, sautéed veggies (request light oil), sashimi-style fish, miso soup, vegetable soup (but watch the sodium), etc. Non-vegetarians can request a simple piece of grilled chicken or fish.

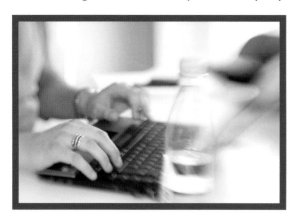

4. *Keep raw nuts, seeds, fruit, and other healthy snacks in your purse, briefcase, or car in case you can't find anything healthy on the menu.*

5. *When traveling, be sure to go online in advance and print out a list of restaurants that serve organic foods, seafood, and "raw" food.*

6. *Take a small ice chest with you whether you are out for the afternoon, the day, the weekend . . . or even on a plane.* Never rely on airline food or airports if you intend to make healthy eating a way of life! My standard "care package" for traveling includes hummus and veggies, raw nuts and seeds, a little fruit, and lean protein or sugar-free protein bars. I also bring my own tea bags and greens for my water. No matter where you are, be sure to have enough food to get you by until you can find the next "healthy meal stop." I carry the same ice chest with me every day when I leave the house.

7. *Once you have arrived and settled in at your destination, make the grocery store your first stop.* Bring a standard list of healthy items with you and stock up on these foods for your trip.

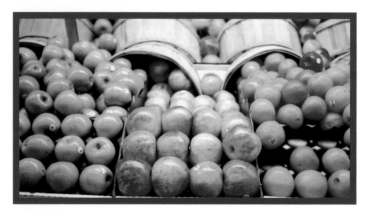

8. *You usually can request a refrigerator in your room if there is not already one there.* Most hotels will accommodate you.

Sometimes, though, our travels take us to places that are literally designed to be a complete escape from day-to-day life and food is integrated into these destinations as part of the overall experience. I used to be a slave to places like Disneyland that don't have my best interest in mind. I made excuses like, "It's only one day" and "You HAVE to blow it when you are at Disneyland!" But, I was tired of feeling guilty and I actually felt tired after days like that. Now I tell myself, "I set the standard for my life" and "I will be a living example of health and fitness!" I do this each time I go out . . . literally every day! It works and it is so much fun to be the creator of my own experiences!

When I recently went to Disneyland for an all-day birthday party, I went with a plan. Places like Disneyland are finally offering some healthier choices. A couple of Disneyland's restaurants offer grilled fish or vegetable and chicken bowls (I don't eat the rice). You also can purchase fruit at one of the many fruit stands around the park. But, Disneyland also has fallen prey to the not-so-healthy "healthy" option phenomena. Read the ingredients on the trail mix at most concession stands and you will see that it contains high fructose corn syrup and sulfur dioxide!

So, I arrived for this party with some organic, raw nuts, and a low-carb protein bar in my makeup bag. When the rest of our group went to the BBQ place to order ribs and fried chicken, I made a beeline for the fruit stand. My lunch consisted of fruit, salad from the restaurant, and nuts. I was prepared! For dessert, I even brought my own sugar-free, raw coconut macaroon and this saved me from the temptation of the assorted cookies, chocolates, and cakes.

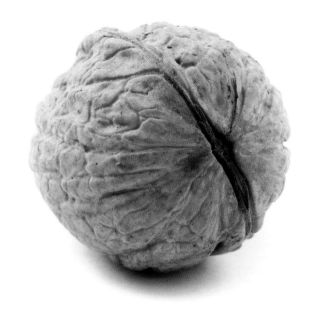

Besides enjoying the fact that I am proactive with my own health, I also enjoy having a positive influence on other people. Several of the women in our group commented that my food plan for that day did not seem all that hard. And, by the end of the day when they all felt awful, I had energy and felt great! The women saw this and started asking me questions. They were ready to listen. I love being in control of my own destiny! And I love helping others realize that they can be too!

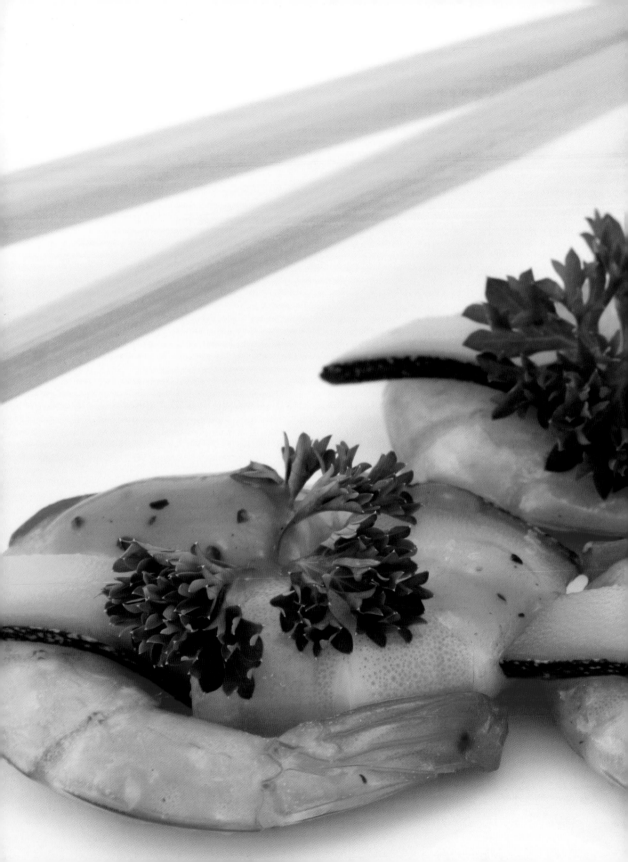

Chapter 7
LET'S PARTY:
Don't Let Party Poopers Rain on Your Parade

Chapter 7

Parties . . . Ah, yes, parties! Parties used to be a major source of stress for me for several reasons. I am Lebanese and I am married to a Lebanese man whose family numbers more people than I collectively know on the planet! If you know anything about Middle Eastern families, then you will know that they love to party and they love to eat. Eating is a way of life, a way of bringing people together and a way of showing love in so many cultures. Most definitely in ours! To show up to someone's home and say you are not eating is taboo. They are either insulted or they walk around trying to stuff food in your face all night while telling you that you are too skinny and need some meat on your bones!

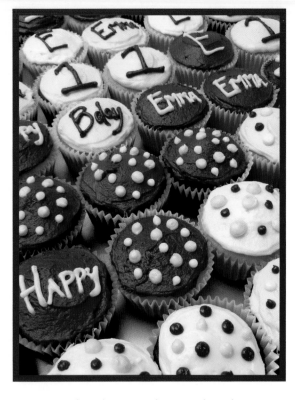

My husband and I eventually were able to get our family to understand and respect the way we eat. But friends may be a different story. It's more difficult to attend parties thrown by friends or business colleagues. You really don't know what you are walking into, and you don't always know everyone as intimately as you do with family. Also, you may not know what foods will be served, and you most likely will not feel comfortable telling these people that you aren't going to eat the amazing rack of lamb with Bordeaux sauce and chocolate soufflé that they spent all day preparing... especially if the hostess is your employer's wife!

Another party problem for me used to be my "sweet tooth." I could manage to follow a healthy eating plan at a party until one of my "trigger" foods was put in front of me. As a result, I found myself either avoiding the parties where I knew these foods would be served or going to the parties and eating these things even though it made me feel awful. Afterwards, I would struggle to get back on track for several days. It was a vicious cycle. Fortunately, I now have kicked my sugar addiction and I no longer am plagued with this issue. However, I do not take anything for granted so I continue to be proactive about my eating. I just do not allow myself to be put into compromising situations without a plan.

Here is my strategy for dealing with my passionate, loving, food-oriented family and friends . . .

1. *Call ahead and find out what is being served so you can be prepared.*

2. *Ask the hostess if they mind if you bring a dish (or two) to accommodate the way you eat.* Most people appreciate the help, and this gives the hostess a "heads up" that you don't eat a typical diet. Again, you are setting an example!

3. *Take a wholesome, healthy dessert with you to the party.* There is an amazing "raw" food restaurant near me that serves the most outrageous desserts. They make them with unprocessed fruit and nuts that haven't had all of the nutrition

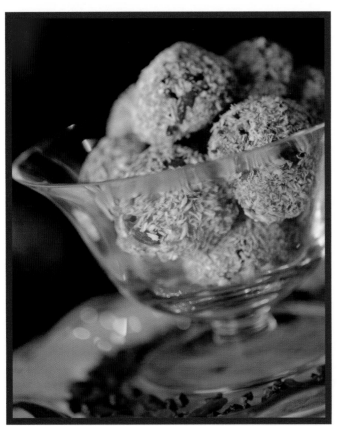

and fiber cooked out of them. The "apple cobbler," "peaches and cream," and "macaroons" are simply decadent. In such places, you even can request that the desserts are made without agave if the restaurant makes their food "to order." While some of these treats are not low in calories and fat (so pay attention), they are raw, living, unprocessed foods that are filled with nutritional value. I find that when I eat a dessert like this—especially after eating a nutritious meal—that I have no desire to gorge the way I would with cake, ice cream, and chips. Fruit does not cause the same biological or psychological reaction, and it leaves you feeling energized and healthy instead.

4. **Carry nuts or seeds with you.**

5. **When attending banquets and functions, eat in advance and then just pick at the veggies and salad.** You can also ask if they are able to accommodate your "health" needs. Many venues now serve grilled fish or

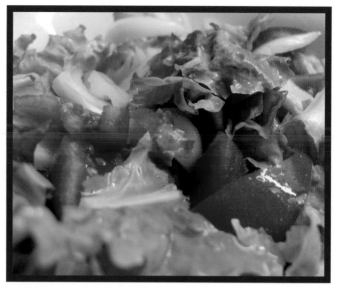

chicken with steamed vegetables for people who have special dietary needs. I often get odd looks when I tell servers that I have "health issues," but they don't argue. Hey, whatever works!

6. Perhaps my biggest tip, though, is something that I have learned from experience. *As I have mentioned several times, you must keep your ice chest in the car and have it filled with your back-up foods.* This way, you can make a quick detour for some healthy snacks that will put an end to your obsession with the Tiramisu. While your brief absence will likely not be noticed by others, this brief departure from the scene can do you a world of good. A change in scenery and some fresh air will do much to alter your state of mind and set your thinking straight. This is called a "pattern interrupt," and it is a very powerful tool. When you are about to "hypnotically" or impulsively fall into a routine behavior, do something to break your regular routine. Go outside and get some air!

Hopefully you are beginning to see a pattern here! Always be prepared and have a plan. Carry that ice chest with your "emergency stash" everywhere you go. If you fail to plan, you plan to fail!

Above all, I have learned that being out and about among people means that you need to understand people . . . and yourself. There are a thousand reasons that people will use to encourage you to join them instead of supporting you on your mission (misery loves company, guilt, "love," companionship, societal conditioning, etc.). This means that you need to be solid in your stand! If you are wishy-washy, people will sense it and be right there to break your stride.

On the contrary, everyone is drawn to a leader. Even if people are uncomfortable and don't agree with you, they will respect your decisions if they sense your conviction. The key is your commitment. And it will be only a short time until people are asking for your advice . . . I promise! So, although there will always will be some "party poopers" around to rain on your parade, you will be surprised at how many people will be supportive of the new stand you take.

Creating Brain Healthy Parties

As I mentioned earlier, being part of a large Lebanese family does not make eating healthy at family gatherings and parties a simple task unless we really set our minds to it. It has traditionally been acceptable to be a little "thick in the middle," and actually considered less attractive to be too thin. When visiting my aunt in Pennsylvania, the first thing I would usually hear upon arriving is, "Oh my! We need to put some weight on you! I have been cooking all weekend. You need to eat." She would stand over me and literally try to put food in my mouth. It was her way of showing love.

If we are going to change the health of our society, we need to change our association to food. We don't need to eliminate our love of gathering, bonding, or even the desire to have food as a central theme. If we put as much energy into creating "brain healthy" choices at our parties and gatherings the outcome would be astounding.

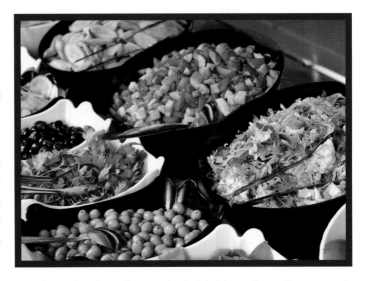

The key is to change your focus and motivation. Instead of thinking about how much you want to impress everyone with your gourmet skills, get clear on what you are really doing and what the real motivation is, or at least could or should be. Be clear that traditional party food and most gourmet foods are filled with fat, salt, sugar, and many other unhealthy ingredients. Start with empowering questions that help to define your goal.

1. *How can I create an outstanding party that will leave my guests even healthier and more energetic?*

2. How can I set an example that being healthy and fit is easy and fun?

Creating brain healthy parties is not very difficult and will eliminate at least some of the pressure and work traditionally associated with the food portion of party planning. Several years a go, I had a surprise birthday party for my husband. I invited more than 100 guests. Knowing that most of the guests would be very health conscious, I knew that I would have to provide at least some of the food myself. However, I also had much of the food catered simply because of the number of people attending. An interesting thing happened.

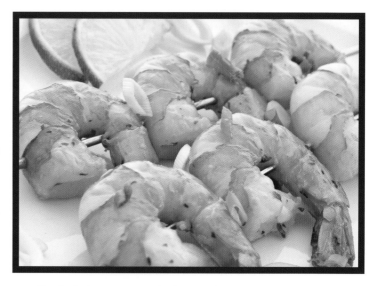

We brought the food out in stages, starting with large platters of fresh fruit and vegetables, accompanied by fresh salsa, guacamole, hummus, baba ghanoush, and non-dairy yogurt dip. There were also bowls of raw nuts sitting around. Along with this course was tabouleh and a cucumber mint salad. The next round of food came about 45 minutes later and included grilled vegetables, artichokes, grilled shrimp, seared ahi, and a couple other things. The least healthy of the food (because of the sauce), was grilled fish, chicken, and pork. I found it fascinating that the meat was all but untouched. Hardly anyone ate it. Although I did serve dessert, again, it was virtually untouched.

As I cleaned up the aftermath of the party, I couldn't help but analyze the remains. The food that I had spent the most money for remained, while the fruit, vegetables, salads, and healthier fare had been devoured. One reason may have been because of an oversight on my part not reminding the catering service to serve the sauces on the side. Or it could have been that the crowd was a fairly health-conscious crowd.

However, I really believe it had more to do with the fact that the guests were offered so many healthy choices to fill up on first! By the time the heavier meats and sauces were brought out the guests had already had time to nibble and graze on fresh, healthy food arranged on beautiful platters.

I learned two very important lessons from this experience.

Lesson One: It doesn't matter how exclusive the guest list is, your guests will appreciate fresh, healthy food that has been beautifully presented. You don't need to spend hundreds or even thousands of dollars on food that will make your guests fat and tired. If you are going to spend the money, spend it on something healthy.

Lesson Two: Bringing food out in courses is a really good idea. Think about it. No matter how beautifully you decorate your house, where do people congregate? The kitchen! We have established that people often gather with food being the central theme. So let them! Bring the food out slowly, in courses. Let your guests graze and nibble slowly. Allow them to fill up on healthy choices prior to serving the main course. You can bet that they will eat smaller portions, which is much healthier.

Even if you are planning a more traditional, sit-down dinner, plan some time in advance for people to visit and munch on healthy appetizers. You don't have to serve traditional, fat-filled dishes. Your main courses can be healthy, creative, and unique.

HELPFUL PARTY TIPS

1. Always serve raw fruits and vegetables first, along with fresh salsa, guacamole, hummus, and baba ghanoush.

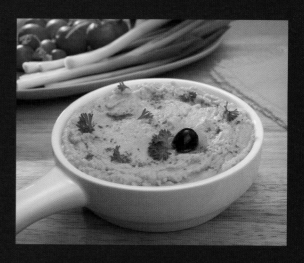

2. Serve flax crackers, gluten-free pita bread or tortillas instead of chips. Baked chips can also be an alternative. Fried chips have acrilomide (a known carcinogen).

3. Next bring out some light and refreshing salads such as the Sassy Cucumber Mint Salad that can be found on page 229 of the *Eat healthy with the Brain Doctor's Wife Cookbook*.

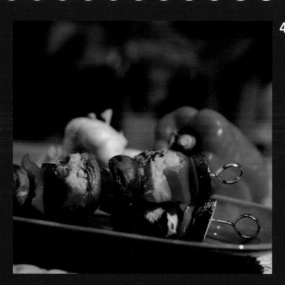

4. **If you are doing the cooking yourself:** Stick to dishes that can be cooked in large portions without much extra effort. Some suggestions: Try grilled vegetables with a light vinaigrette sauce, grilled fish, or kabobs. If you are serving chicken, fish, or kabobs of any kind, preparation can be done well in advance so that you only need to spend a few minutes grilling.

5. **If you are planning to use a caterer:** Make sure you understand what the ingredients are in the sauces they are serving. Do not trust them if they tell you they are "light" and "everyone likes them." Have them serve all sauces on the side. If you are serving food in the fashion mentioned above, you will likely not need as much food as you think you will. I can easily order main courses for half the number of guests. Most of the guests do not take as large a portion as is normally served. I still usually end up with lots of excess food.

6. **End with something fresh and light for dessert.** Your guests won't miss the flourless chocolate cake. If you really want to have something decadent, try putting out a bowl of "healthy" chocolates. There are a couple brands of dark chocolate that are sweetened with fruit juice or acai berries. One brand has an ORAC value of over 11,000 and has very little caffeine.

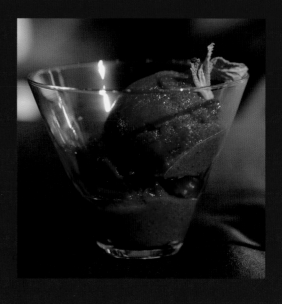

7. Know your guest list well. Be aware of any special dietary needs of guests. Know if there is a guest who is diabetic or if you will be having guests who are vegan (vegans do not consume any animal products, including eggs, dairy, or honey). Vegan diets are becoming increasingly popular. It is a good idea to provide a menu healthy enough to feed either of these dietary needs. Have at least a couple of tasty options available.

8. Do not be afraid to ask for help from close friends and family. One of the greatest things about marrying into my new family is the abundance of love and help at my fingertips at any given time. While it was difficult for me to ask for help initially, I found that when I did it created a stronger sense of family... for me! My new family gladly helped, and they began to bond with me. As I said, Middle Eastern families love to gather around food. It's likely that you will find some of the people in your own circles who feel the same. It is a party after all.

BRAIN HEALTHY PARTY FOODS

Hosting a party with brain healthy fare is easy. The tasty finger foods listed here include many of the 50 Best Brain Foods and Brain Healthy Spices—you'll find these brain-enhancing foods and spices in bold. Packed with potent antioxidants and nutrients, these party foods will boost brain function for an unforgettable soirée.

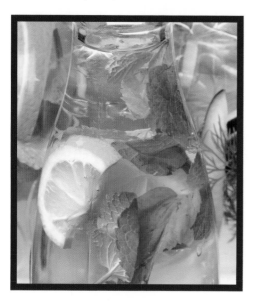

- **Holiday Spiced Green Tea: Mix green tea leaves with chopped and dried orange peel, chopped and dried ginger root, and cinnamon. Add unsweetened almond milk for a healthy version of a chai tea. Consider cinnamon-flavored stevia as a sweetener if desired.**

- **Spa Water: Serve sparkling or flat water with lemon or lime wedges. Lemon-flavored stevia makes this taste like lemonade... even children love it.**

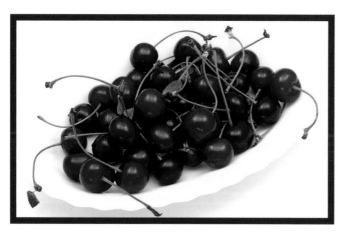

- **Raw Veggies Tray:** You can include broccoli florets; red, yellow, orange, and green bell peppers; cherry tomatoes; and carrots.

- **Fruit Bowl**

- **Fill a bowl with cherries**

- **Hummus:** Made from garbanzo beans, lemon juice, tahini, olive oil, and garlic.

- **Guacamole:** Mix avocado with onions, tomatoes, serrano chiles, and lime or lemon juice.

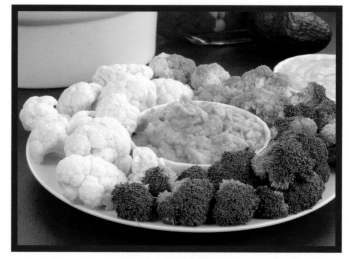

- **Salsa:** Combine tomatoes, onions, cilantro, jalapeno peppers, lime, garlic powder, cumin (found in curry).

- **Black Bean Dip:** Purée black beans, red onion, orange or lime juice, cilantro, olive oil, garlic, and cumin (found in curry) in a blender.

- **Bruschetta:** Try using gluten-free, flourless bread (Ezekiel) or raw flax crackers instead of white bread and top with heirloom tomatoes, a little olive oil, and lots of fresh basil.

- **Shrimp Kebabs:** Marinate shrimp in olive oil, garlic, and lemon.

- **Chicken Skewers:** Grill chicken breasts marinated in plain coconut milk yogurt, curry, fresh ginger, and garlic.

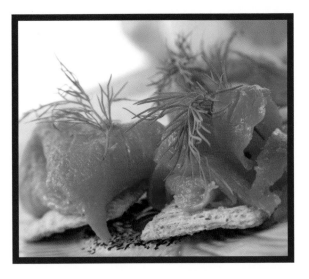

- **Smoked Wild Salmon:** Serve smoked wild salmon with lemon, capers, and dill on gluten free, flourless bread (Ezekiel) or raw flax crackers.

- **Yogurt Parfait:** Top plain Greek yogurt (or non-dairy coconut milk yogurt with live cultures) with blueberries, strawberries, and raspberries, then sprinkle with chopped almonds for a tasty dessert.

- **Shrimp Cocktail:** Serve jumbo shrimp with homemade cocktail sauce made with salsa, horseradish, and lemon juice. Be sure to check ingredients on horseradish for HFCS, MSG, and other hidden, health destroying ingredients.

- **Sashimi Rolls:** Roll sushi-grade wild salmon or tuna with avocado, cucumber, and asparagus then wrap with seaweed.

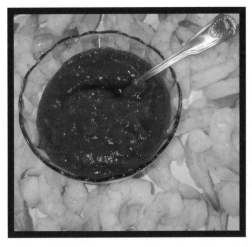

- **Edamame:** Cooked soybeans go great with sushi.

- **Mixed Nuts:** Can include walnuts, almonds, cashews, and pecans, preferably raw — roasting nuts eliminates most of the nutritional value and leaves you with the bad fat and salt.

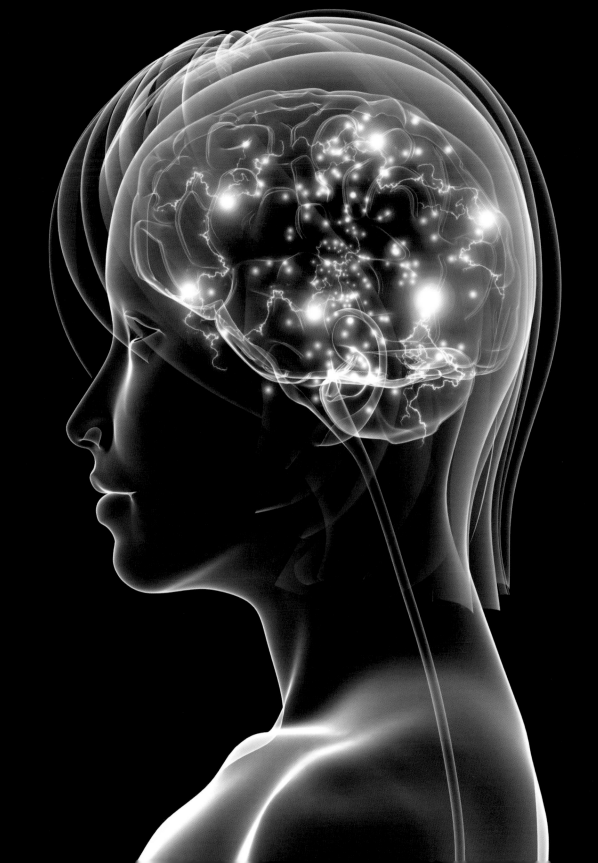

Chapter 8

GET YOUR MIND RIGHT: Your "Hardware" and "Software" Need to Run in Harmony

Chapter 8

GET YOUR MIND RIGHT: Your "Hardware" and "Software" Need to Run in Harmony

Did you know that only a very small part of the success of any major decision is based on hard work and willpower? Often times, the harder you work, the harder the task becomes and the more likely you are to fail. When it comes to success—whether in weight loss, in changing your lifestyle, in work, in relationships, etc.—how you think may be more important than what you do! Your brain is more complex than the most sophisticated, powerful computer ever created.

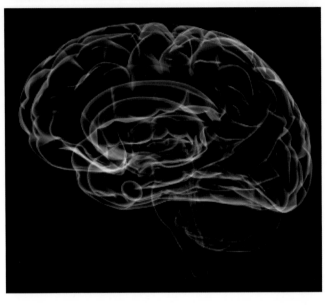

Think of your psychology as the "software" for this computer. This is the set of beliefs and meanings that you hold in your mind. It is what you input into your "hardware." The "hardware" is your biology, your brain function. Both this "software" and this "hardware" have to be working properly, and in harmony, for you to succeed. In other words, your brain must be both physically and mentally healthy for you to most easily achieve success.

When it comes to weight loss and lifestyle change, having this "software" and "hardware" running in synch will mean that following a health-promoting plan won't be "hard work." After all, if you are finally giving your body the fuel that it thrives on and is designed for, your "hardware" will be functioning at its optimal levels. Then, if you reprogram your "software" with a health-promoting psychology, your new adventure in wellness can be fun and exciting rather than difficult and daunting!

But how do you reprogram your "software?" First, you must educate yourself about the proper way to eat so that you can unleash your metabolism! This book is one tool for taking this necessary step. Second, you must educate yourself about your own body and your own health. Third, you must enlist the help of other people who can serve as mentors and companions on your journey. Fourth, you must make your "software" healthy by doing the proper exercises. ***That's right - you can exercise your psychology!***

"Fat Thinking" vs. "Fit Thinking"

After interviewing many clients, both overweight and fit, I began to realize that there are some powerful distinctions in how they think about their weight and their health.

When fit clients were asked how they would feel if they were to become fat and couldn't work out, they had similar responses. Here is a summary of those responses:

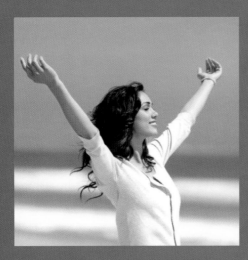

- Fit clients could not and would not imagine being fat.

- Fit people use different physiology, meaning they stand and talk differently than their unfit peers.

- Most said they experience physical discomfort (shortness of breath, achy joints, etc.) when they are only a few pounds over their ideal weight.

- Many said they have trouble sleeping at night and that they are disturbed by the "feeling of fat" on their bodies even if they are only 2 or 3 pounds over their ideal weight!

- Nearly all concurred that they would find a way to work out even if they were confined to a wheelchair!

When overweight, unfit clients were asked how they would feel if they were fit, healthy, and at an ideal weight, they had similar responses as well. Here is a summary of those responses:

- Nearly all believed that they are genetically destined to be fat. Only one said she is lazy.

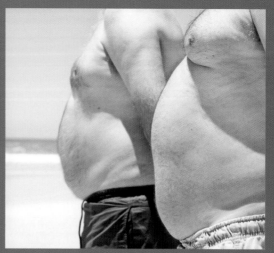

- Most said they couldn't really picture being fit even though they had tried many extreme fad diets and had lost (but then gained) significant amounts of weight.

- They all had numerous excuses for why they could not lose weight including expense, time commitment, "too boring," "too difficult," etc.

- They all agreed that they lacked energy.

With the general beliefs held by the "fit" group, how likely do you think it is that any of these people will ever be fat (as long as their internal picture doesn't change)? They are all completely dedicated to doing whatever it takes to stay fit and healthy. Being overweight is not even conceivable to this group!

On the other hand, our "unfit" group has some major reprogramming of their "software" to do if they ever intend to experience the long-term benefits of health and fitness. If you can't see it, you can't achieve it . . . at least not permanently. This is at least part of the reason why people who are overweight yo-yo diet and continuously lose then regain the weight. Their "software" is telling them that they are destined to be overweight and unhealthy.

This may sound like a harsh generalization. I realize that life doesn't occur in a bubble. I was overweight and depressed when I had thyroid cancer. Sometimes life throws us some wicked curveballs. But I also know from first-hand experience that, with few exceptions, there is always a solution. You just need to reprogram your "software" so that you can begin the process of finding and applying this solution. It is my passion in life to help people find these solutions through education. This book discusses in detail how to get your "hardware" healthy. Now you need to get your "software" healthy so it can run in harmony with your "hardware." In doing so, you will experience the true joy and passion that you were created for!

Synchronizing Your Software With Your Hardware

1. **Meditation and Prayer:** These are two of the most powerful tools you have at your disposal and they are free! Someone once explained the difference to me by saying that prayer is the act of talking to God and meditation is the act of listening. Studies have shown that prayer and meditation actually activate the front part of the

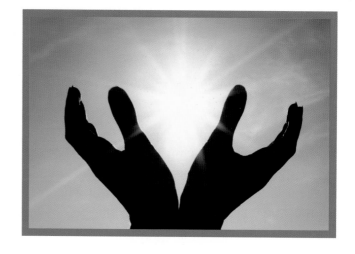

brain. This is the portion of the brain that is responsible for judgment, forethought, and impulse control. Just set aside five or 10 minutes, first thing in the morning, for mediation and/or prayer.

2. **Gratitude:** Start every day by journaling five things for which you are grateful. This actually alters brain chemistry!

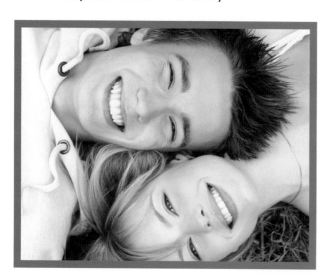

3. **Focus:** "Where your focus goes, your energy flows." — Anthony Robbins. Focus on how awful it feels to be unfit while simultaneously focusing on the amazing benefits that you are going to gain from your new lifestyle. Focus on the increased energy, vitality, improved sleep, and enhanced love life you are going to experience.

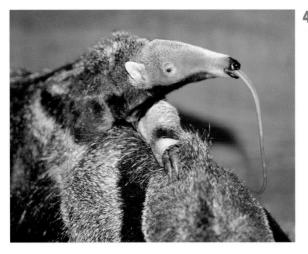

4. **ANTeater:** Pay attention to your "Automatic Negative Thoughts" (ANTs) and develop an "ANTeater." Some of my favorite tips for dealing with those pesky negative thoughts are explained by my husband in his book *The Amen Solution*. Author of the bestselling book *Loving What Is*, Byron Katie also deals with this in *The Work of Byron Katie*. You can download free worksheets from www.thework.com.

5. **Visual Aids:** People will go to greater lengths to avoid pain than to gain pleasure. For this reason, you must utilize both positive and negative reinforcements. Look at photos of someone with your ideal body (maybe even you at another time in your life) and look at photos of you when you feel miserable and unfit. But you must be realistic—don't choose photos of some anorexic model!

6. **Journaling:** Keep a "food diary." Journaling your food will help to keep you on track. You will notice the foods that you eat unconsciously and that are sabotaging your success.

7. **"Hardware" Check:** Make certain that your brain is functioning correctly. Know your brain type and your relevant medical numbers such as vitamin D, thyroid, cholesterol, blood pressure, hormones, etc. You can find a list of relevant numbers in appendix 2. In addition, you can fill out a questionnaire to determine your brain type online at www.amenclinics.com.

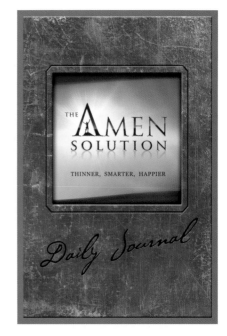

8. **Trauma:** Deal with past emotional trauma through the guidance of a trained professional. Emotional trauma can have a major negative impact on your health goals and even on your weight due to increased stress hormones and other chemicals. These hormones also increase the incidence of depression.

9. Mentors: Most successful people I know have a mentor. There is no reason to reinvent the wheel! Also, this will increase your accountability while making the journey a lot more fun.

Beyond these steps, you can begin to reprogram your "software" by engaging in a powerful exercise that is known as "Bridging." This exercise is a highly valuable tool for helping you to change your internal picture of yourself. Take 30 minutes, get out some paper and a pencil, put on some motivating music, and really get into it.

BRIDGING EXERCISE

- Who will I be in 10 Years ideally?

- Describe in detail who you want to be in 10 years?

- How do you look?

- What are you wearing?

- Who are you with?

- Are you laughing, crying, happy, ecstatic?

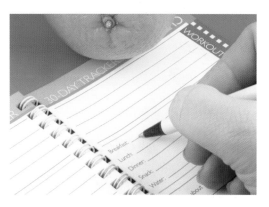

- What is your daily routine?

- What do you do for exercise?

- How much energy do you have?

- What is your posture like?

- What do you like to eat?

- What do you do for fun?

- What is your health like?

- What do other people think of you?

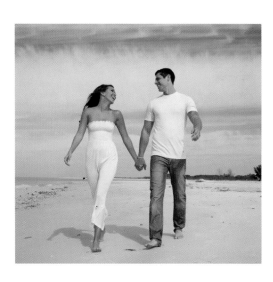

- Who are you an inspiration for?

- If you were able to meet this "ideal" you, what questions would you ask him/her that would help you to succeed in achieving this "ideal?"

Who will I be in five years . . . Ideally? (Repeat the same process by answering the same questions.)

Who will I be in one year . . . Ideally? (Repeat the same process by answering the same questions.)

Who will I be in six months, three months, one month, one week . . . Ideally? (Repeat the same process.)

Final Step:

Go back through what you have written. Everywhere that you have written "I will be," change it to "I am." Read it through after this and really feel it, really own it. Begin to think it and live it!

I suggest making a copy of it and carrying it with you. Put another copy up where you will see it often. Read it as often as possible. Keeping it around you all the time will exert an influence on you even when you are not reading it. Allow this process to begin to manifest amazing results in your life and in the lives of everyone you care about!

A Note About "Listening" ...

For my busy brain, "talking to God" was a lot easier than passively "listening." And, frankly, I didn't think it was that big of a deal for me. Since I pray, visualize, work out, and do so many other things for my health, I figured I could skip this one. Even though I knew that it would be good for me, I found every excuse not to do it.

But, the world works in mysterious ways. A while back I decided to organize a self-defense class for the ladies in my neighborhood. A friend of mine who is a Los Angeles Police Department "Special Weapons And Tactics" officer taught the class. Of all the people who had been telling me that I would really benefit from meditation, he was not a person that I expected to hear it from too! What does a macho SWAT cop know about meditation? A great deal, it turns out!

In the short time that we trained together, he told me several times that I would benefit from taking five minutes each morning to quiet my mind. I told him that I didn't have the time. Well... he used the same line on me that I use on everyone else! He said, "As hectic as your life is, you don't have time not to meditate! If we looked at your life on paper, I bet that you don't have time to work out either, but you do it! But meditating is probably one of the most important things you can do for yourself."

I must say, he was right. It has been a great investment. I have gained more mental clarity, focus, and creativity since I began meditating. And, maybe it's just my imagination, but really nice, positive "coincidences" began happening since then as well!

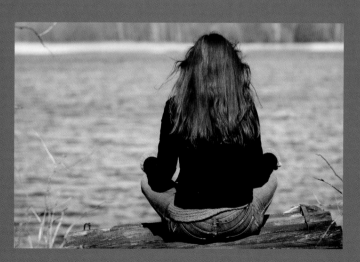

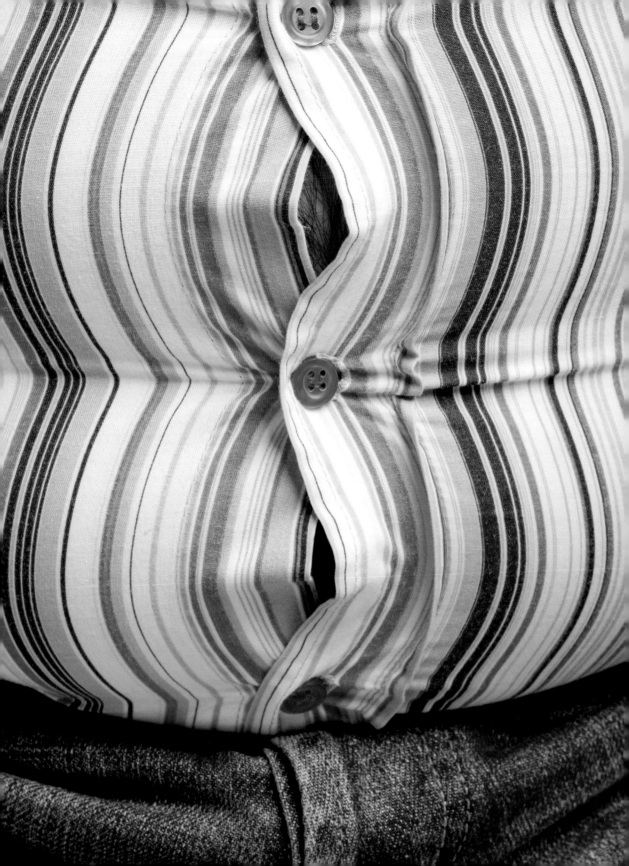

Chapter 9

THE "BIG" PICTURE AIN'T SO PRETTY: Obesity and Other Eating Disorders

Chapter 9

||||||||||||||||||||||||||||||||||||||||||||||||||||||||||||||||||||||||||||||||||||||||||||||||||||||||||||||||||||||||||||||

THE "BIG" PICTURE AIN'T SO PRETTY:
Obesity and Other Eating Disorders

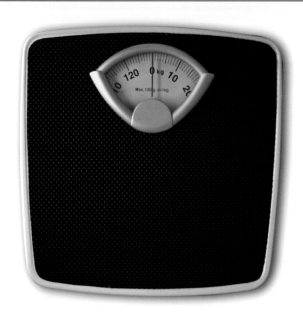

Every day we are bombarded by conflicting messages about weight. On the one hand, we hear about "The Fat Movement" which expounds the rights of people to be as fat as they wish without being discriminated against. The food industry, of course, backs this movement while simultaneously "supersizing" everything we eat! On the other hand, we have the media and the fashion industry giving only the most anorexic of the bunch the opportunity to grace our televisions, movie screens, and fashion magazines. They do this while sacrificing the health, the well-being, and sometimes the lives of those people they have thrust to the forefront. As a result, the issues of weight and food have become highly complex, controversial, and confusing in our society.

However, it doesn't take a genius to look around and see that we have a rapidly growing problem on our hands—literally. From 1980 to 2007, the number of Americans with Type 2 Diabetes tripled. And, according to the Centers for Disease Control, an estimated 7 million Americans are walking around with diabetes right now and they don't even know it! It is no wonder that the U.S. spends approximately $132 billion each year on diabetes.

Our society's unhealthy relationship with food and weight also makes it impossible to write about food and nutrition without mentioning the elephant in the room . . . Eating Disorders. It's actually very difficult to talk about weight and nutrition without offending someone. If you know anyone with an eating disorder—obesity included—then you know what I am talking about firsthand.

For people dealing with disordered eating, food becomes an obsession and takes on a life of its own. These people have an ambivalent relationship with food at best. Food is their "enemy" or food is their "best friend" rather than being the fuel it is intended to be. Food has perceived power over them. From the moment they wake up they are consumed with thoughts of how they will "deal with food." They often experience denial about their relationship with food. This is because they "dissociate"—not in the sense of a split personality, but as a way to desensitize feelings that are just too difficult or too painful to process.

- **Nearly 24 million Americans suffer from an eating disorder in some form.**

- **Nearly one in five women struggle with an eating disorder in some form.**

- **Recent studies show "Binge Eating" to be the most common form of disordered eating.**

- **Eating disorders continue to have the highest mortality rate of any mental health illness!**

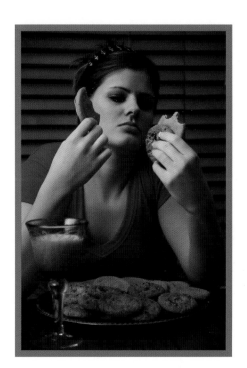

Obesity-Related Illnesses

- **Cardiovascular Disease**
- **Atherosclerosis**
- **Stroke**
- **High Blood Pressure**

- **Gout**
- **Gallstones**
- **Other Eating Disorders**

A Note about Obesity and Cancer . . .

Most people are aware that obesity is linked directly to heart disease, high blood pressure, gout, gallstones, and stroke, but many people are not as aware that obesity also is linked to many types of cancers; And being overweight doesn't just increase your chances of developing certain cancers; being overweight also increases the chances that you will die of cancer! This may be a function of being overweight. But, it also may be a result of the typical high-calorie, high-fat, low-fiber diet that most overweight people consume. Obese women are most at risk for developing uterine, gallbladder, ovarian, breast, and colon cancer. Obese men are most at risk for developing colorectal and prostate cancer.

This less-publicized danger also highlights the greatest danger that exists for people who suffer from eating disorders—the lack of truly informed, widely disseminated, factual, and useful information about these terrible problems. For instance, I am certain that you have heard of obesity, but you may never have heard of "Compulsive Overeaters." Likewise, I am certain that you have heard of anorexia and bulimia, but you may never have heard that young women are not the only people affected by these terrible conditions. Finally, I am certain that although you "know" about eating disorders, you may not know what to do about them!

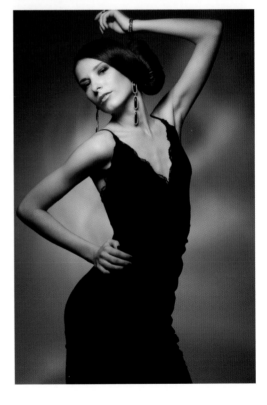

With the exception of obesity, it is hard to know who has an eating disorder. Anorexia becomes obvious to the outside observer, but it does not start out that way. Bulimia is even trickier, as people suffering from this disorder are usually close to "normal" weight. People who are purging by vomiting, taking laxatives, and/or engaging in extreme exercise, may not exhibit symptoms to the casual or uninformed observer. This is further complicated by the fact that these people tend to be such perfectionists that they will guard their "loathsome secret" that much tighter. It is estimated that only one-third of people with anorexia and only 6 percent of people with bulimia ever receive care, which makes accurate reporting nearly impossible.

Sadly, more and more young males also succumb to eating disorders. They feel tremendous pressure about their physiques. This pressure is compounded by the fact that a diet filled with refined carbohydrates, fast foods, cheap oils, and sugar triggers impulsivity, diminishes energy, and causes a continual battle of the bulge. No one—not even young men—can maintain an extremely lean physique with this kind of diet. Yet, our society values a perfect, ultra-lean physique in young men. This creates the perfect storm for eating disorders.

Her daily diet... Right?!

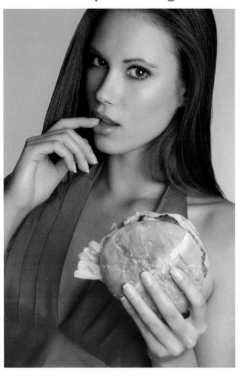

Likewise, middle-aged women make up a fairly significant, but discreet, population of people who are suffering with bulimia and anorexia. It is difficult to know just how many women struggle with these life-threatening disorders. Experts believe that any numbers that can be compiled need to be adjusted even higher because shame and stigma prevent women from reporting their disorders. These women tend not to get help until they are experiencing life-threatening symptoms.

Despite this lack of reporting, experts have been able to discern a number of reasons why middle-age women represent a growing percentage of the population of people who suffer from disordered eating. These reasons are:

- **A lack of coping skills**

- **Marital problems and divorce**

- **Empty-Nest syndrome**

- **Societal pressures: "40 is the new 20!"**

- **Hormonal imbalances**

- **Chemical imbalances**

- **Lousy nutrition, leading to hormonal and chemical imbalances!**

- **Unresolved trauma**

- **Major life stressors and the changes that occur at this stage in life**

In addition, the following is a list of the most common contributing factors related to disordered eating behaviors of all kinds and in all eating disorder populations:

- *Hormonal Influences:* Thyroid problems and elevated cortisol indicate chronic stress. Leptin and ghrelin imbalances compromise the hunger and satiety response.

- *Brain Imbalances:* Neurotransmitters such as dopamine and serotonin can wreak havoc on your appetite centers if they are out of balance.

- *ADD or Head Injuries:* These affect the activity in the frontal lobes and lead to lowered inhibitions, decreased judgment, elevated impulsivity, compulsivity, and obsessiveness.

- *Genetic Influences:* Researchers have identified specific chromosomes that are believed to be associated with bulimia and anorexia.

- *Societal and Age-Related Influences:* Unrealistic photos and media messages abound alongside ads for the sale of processed foods and "supersizing."

- *Past Emotional Traumas*

Signs and Symptoms of Eating Disorders

Compulsive Overeating:

- Dramatic weight gain in a short period of time

- Chronic yo-yo dieting

- Mood swings and depression

- Chronic fatigue

- Elevated blood pressure and cholesterol

- Doesn't stop eating even when full

- Fear of loss of control over food

- Blames weight for not having the life they want

- Believes that food is the "drug" that makes everything all right

- Talks about food like it's a friend . . . or an enemy

- Hides food in strange places

Bulimia and Anorexia:

- Obsession with weight, even when underweight or at normal weight

- Food is hidden to avoid eating it

- Money is spent in excessive amounts for food (during binging)

- Unusual food rituals

- Self-starvation

- Frequent visits to the restroom shortly after a meal

- Knuckles are bruised and/or teeth are eroded

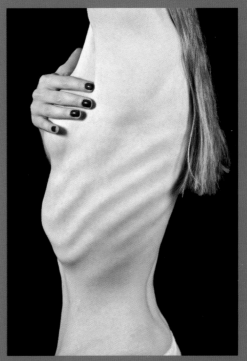

- Dizziness

- Irregular heart beat and heart rate due to electrolyte imbalance

- Loss of hair

- Lanugo (fine baby hair covering the body)

- Loss of menstruation

- Radical mood swings, depression

- Chronic fatigue

- Insomnia

- Perfectionism and self-criticism

- Self-esteem is low

- Inability to show intimacy, yet often promiscuous

- Self-imposed isolation so they won't be "found out"

Though we do know the signs, symptoms and common features of disordered eating, it is still difficult to know if eating disorders are:

1. **Fueled by an underlying medical, hormonal, or brain issue, or**

2. **If medical and brain issues are being fueled by the disordered eating behavior.**

Either way, eating disorders create a vicious circle that is nearly impossible for most people to break away from without the help of a qualified professional. Effectively treating disordered eating behaviors requires the help of a trained professional who will treat patients from a bio-psycho-social-spiritual perspective. If you know someone who is engaging in this deadly behavior, do all that you can to get them help immediately—you might just save this person's life!

In addition to seeking immediate and specific medical intervention, my husband has recommended the following as powerful tools for addressing disordered eating:

*   Eye Movement Desensitization and Reprocessing (EMDR): This is an excellent method for helping patients to process past trauma and for helping patients with post-traumatic stress disorder.

*   Hypnosis

*   Meditation and prayer

*   "The Work" of Byron Katie: Dr. Amen often refers to this as a simple and elegant form of cognitive therapy. It is based upon four simple questions that can be found both in her book *Loving What Is* and on her website www.thework.com.

A Note about "Eating Disorders" versus "Thinking Disorders"...

Several years ago I accompanied my husband to a seminar led by a dear friend of his, Byron Katie. She also goes by Katie. I knew little of her at the time other than that she is a writer and a speaker who attracts a "spiritual" crowd of people who are trying to better themselves in some way or another. Many of the people who follow her work are struggling with addictions. She is not a doctor, nor does she make any medical claims. The people who come to her are a more "earthy" kind of crowd. When I did meet her, I realized that Katie is an ethereal sort of person who is beautiful and gentle from the inside out.

And there I was—an intense, martial-arts-practicing trauma nurse. Let's just say I had a lot to learn! I felt like a fish out of water in my designer jeans while everyone else shuffled in wearing yoga pants and eating tofu! In fact, this "seminar" actually was more of a free-form gathering. It was not specifically about addictions or eating disorders, but that's the direction it quickly took.

Katie asked us to do an exercise in which we all wrote down everything we hated about our bodies, no matter how trivial. This was easy for me. As a perfectionist, I was used to finding the negative in myself. Within a matter of minutes I had a healthy-sized list. As I was kicking back on my yoga mat with my eyes closed, Katie asked for a volunteer to read her list. I could hear the volunteer's voice, but I couldn't see her. I was struck by her words. Her list was nearly identical to mine!

But, by her voice, I knew that she was heavy. I opened my eyes and looked around. The woman who was speaking was at least 15 years older than me and she must have weighed nearly 300 pounds. How was it possible that we had nearly the same list of things that we hated about our bodies? This went on through several more women. Guess what? There was very little difference in any of our lists! Me, obsessive about exercise and in my size 2 jeans, 20-year-old women with anorexia, 300-pound women in their 50s. We all hated the same things about our bodies. You know why?

- *Because our bodies aren't perfect.*

- *Because "disordered thinking" is even more prevalent than disordered eating... one fuels the other.*

- *Because society has planted an ideal of perfectionism that is impossible to achieve.*

- *Because we are human. * Grace goes a long way in healing human imperfection.*

Food is fuel for your body. It has only the power that you give it. It's time that you take your power back and begin using food the way it is intended.

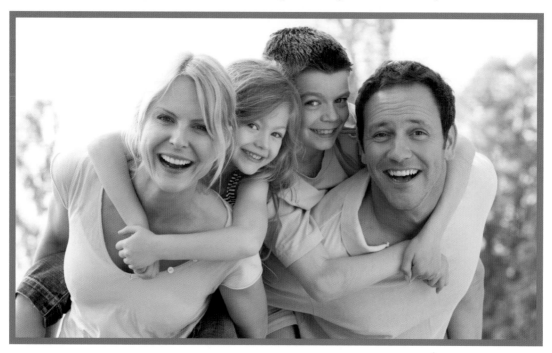

We absolutely must improve our relationship with food. We need to do this for ourselves. But, even more important, we need to do this for our children.

1. 17 percent of American adolescents are obese . . . not a little overweight, obese!

2. 10 percent of preschoolers are more overweight than what is healthy for them!

3. 80 percent of children who are overweight become overweight adults. It's a widely known fact that obesity is one of the leading, preventable burdens to our health system... leading to Type 2 Diabetes, heart disease, and cancer. If your children are obese, they are being set up for a dismal future.

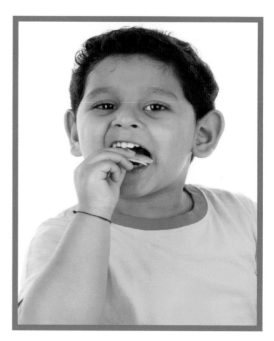

4. Bulimic and anorexic behaviors typically start around puberty. The popular website www.bulimiahelp.org reports that 12 to 14 is the most common age group to experience the onset of these eating disorders.

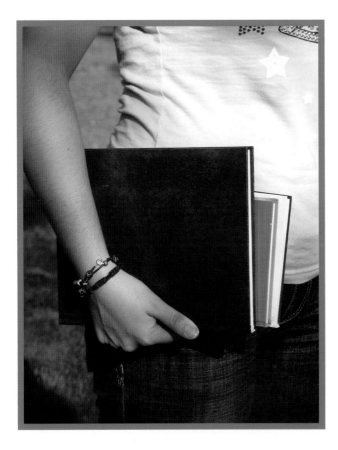

5. It is estimated that up to 30 percent of college-aged women experience disordered eating behaviors at some time during their college careers.

6. Up to 10 percent of nine-year-olds surveyed have reported trying to vomit their food at least one time after feeling that they had eaten too much. Half of them admitted to being on a diet at one time or to dieting regularly because they think they are fat.

7. A maternal history of eating disorders is often a factor for young girls.

8. Most young girls start dieting at the urging of their mothers.

Ultimately, children will make their own choices. You have a limited opportunity to influence your children and educate them when they are young. The best way to do this is through example. Start now!

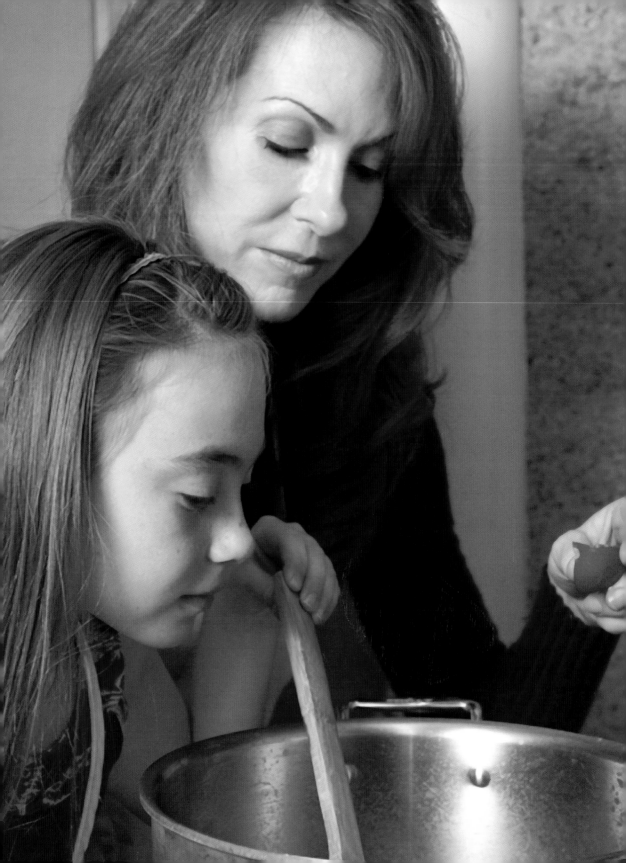

Chapter 10

BUT MY KIDS WILL ONLY EAT POP-TARTS & PIZZA! Get Your Kids Involved Early

BUT MY KIDS WILL ONLY EAT POP-TARTS AND PIZZA!
Get Your Kids Involved Early

"Exposure equals preference." — JJ Virgin

My husband and I got used to the snickers and smiles we would get from people when they would see our daughter, Chloe, eating salmon and avocado at age three. We've long been accustomed to hearing comments from other parents when they see her snacking on red bell peppers and hummus in the airport. Most often, these parents just want to know how we got our strong-willed child to eat anything other than fast food and juice! Simply stated, it has never been an option. When she was really little we didn't provide food for her that we did not want her to have. As a result, she never developed the taste for it or the tendency to reach for it!

Of course, Chloe doesn't live in a bubble. Nor do we want her to. She is a normal seven-year-old and she loves the same things all kids love. If I had cake and ice cream in the house all the time, she would be eating it on a regular basis within a matter of weeks. Also, now that she is a little older, she does see the different foods and ways of eat-

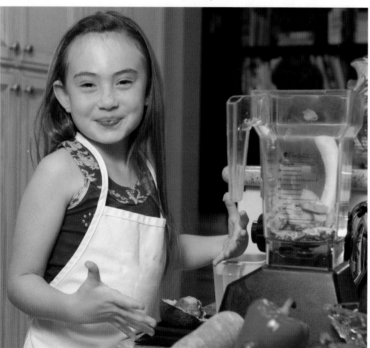

ing that are so prevalent in our society. But because I don't have unhealthy food in the house and I have fresh fruit and vegetables instead, Chloe has learned to enjoy this way of eating. "Exposure equals preference!"

Just as importantly, we have always taught Chloe to make healthy decisions for herself. It is her natural tendency to reach for healthy, nutritious, and energizing foods, but we have never forced her to make these choices. Forcing the matter only causes children to develop the same issues about food that many of you may have . . . the same ones that may have lead you to purchase this book. And let's face it, you can't be with them 24/7. It is far more effective to teach, guide, and empower them to make the healthiest choices possible for themselves! Help your children develop a connection with their bodies, an awareness of how food affects them, and a sense of how food makes them feel.

I often am overjoyed by the choices my daughter makes about food, even when she was as young as five and six years old. Her wisdom and ability to listen to her body already far surpass what it took me decades to accomplish! Once, when I was volunteering at Chloe's school on Halloween, I was put in charge of helping the children decorate cookies . . . with icing! When they were finished, the children were allowed to choose one cookie to take to lunch with them. Most of the children were trying to take more than one. Chloe refused to take her cookie. Her teacher told her three times to get a cookie, but she refused. Figuring it was because I was in the room, I told her that she could have a cookie. Chloe responded, "I don't want a cookie now. It will make my tummy hurt and I will feel sick. I will take it home and eat it after dinner if I want it."

I was happy for several reasons.

1. *Chloe clearly understood how the cookie would affect her body.*

2. *She listened to her body.*

3. *She did not give in to "group think" and, instead, stood on her own.*

4. *She did not allow anyone to influence her when she knew something wasn't good for her—not even a figure of authority.*

Of course, this is not easy for any child. I get so frustrated when I take my daughter to church or school and discover that they have given cookies and candy to the kids without asking the parents. These are places that I trust to be teaching our children, not making them unhealthy. If our children are rewarded with junk food, it doesn't take long for them to develop a very positive association with . . . junk food! This is not what I want to teach my daughter! And we wonder why we have an epidemic of obese and behaviorally disordered children?

People often criticize my intensity on this subject because, after all, it's "only one doughnut." But all of those single doughnuts add up . . . and your kids end up developing a sugar addiction. Why can't we give the kids grapes or strawberries instead?

We have Chloe convinced that blueberries are "God's Candy." *I believe that it isn't possible to be too passionate about having our children eat in a healthy way. There is nothing more important than our children's health!*

Brain Healthy Tips for Kids

- Only keep healthy foods in the house.

- All foods that kids have access to should be nutritious and energizing.

- Don't have any foods that are "taboo" . . . just get rid of them!

- When kids are small, place "parent-approved" items on a "snack shelf" that they can reach.

- Food should be a good experience for kids.

- Play games with kids to help them understand how food affects their bodies and brains.

- Teach your kids about the specific effects of certain foods or ingredients (such as sugar, red dye, MSG, etc.) as early as possible. Let them know what foods contain these substances.

- Teach them to be responsible for their own nutrition as early as possible . . . at school, church, birthday parties, etc.

Of course, all of this is easier if your children are still young and you are in complete control of the shopping and of what they eat. If you have older children and you are just beginning your journey into a lifestyle of healthy eating, this may be a bit more challenging. But, there are some steps that you can take to put them on the path to a life of healthy eating.

1. *Leading by example is the best thing you can do.*

2. *Do not have junk food around the house.*

3. *Do not force them to eat foods that they hate and do not be mean about food.* If you become the "food police," then your children will resent the changes that you are making.

4. Introduce several new healthy dishes each week but also continue to serve one or two of their familiar foods (the healthiest of them). When doing this, quickly eliminate the worst things that they eat then slowly begin eliminating the other less-than-ideal foods. Work towards replacing these foods with more wholesome choices like fruit, salads, soups, smoothies, "raw" homemade desserts, etc.

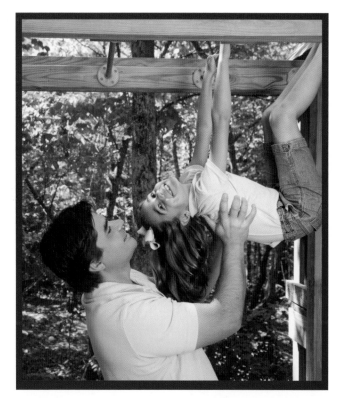

There is no doubt that all of this requires effort, time, patience, and persistence. Yet it will be worth it in the end. Just look around and you will see that we live in a society that is seeped in "food issues" and that these issues are afflicting our little ones. Childhood obesity is increasing at alarming rates, and it is estimated that one out of every three children born after the year 2000 will end up with Type 2 Diabetes.

In our society, we look to food for comfort, fun, love, relief . . . well, for almost everything. We already have discussed the physiology of what happens when your hunger/satiety hormonal system melts down from eating the wrong combination of foods. But if you develop an unhealthy relationship with food and learn to use food for comfort, reward, or punishment, this becomes a psychological issue and not just a hormonal one. Your hunger/satiety balance can be compromised by your psychology. It is very important to remain firmly rooted to the "mind-body" connection during early development and to learn to listen to the signals your body is sending as it relates to hunger, fullness, and how different foods make you feel.

Helping Kids Develop a Healthy Relationship with Food

- Focus on health risk and reward . . . not physical appearance!

- Teach about healthy eating and nutrition, not dieting . . . ever!

- Help kids make connections to how they feel and what they eat. When they eat nutritious food ask them how they feel. Help them to give these feelings a name, "energized," etc. When they eat sugar, point out when they "are more hyper" or when they "get a time out more often."

- Allow kids to experience consequences for the choices they make. If they make less healthy choices, don't nag them but be clear about why they may have a "tummy ache."

- Never make children eat when they are not hungry (unless there is a medical reason for doing so).

- Avoid using food as reward.

- Avoid using food as punishment.

- Don't allow sugary desserts if children choose not to eat . . . give them back their nutritious meal to eat first.

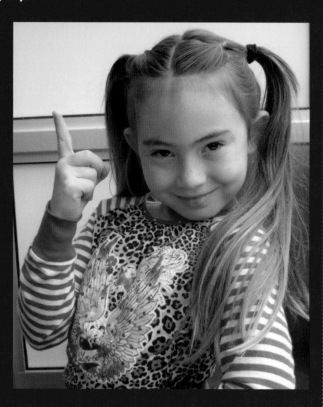

- Get kids involved in cooking early . . . and make it fun!

- Emphasize that food is fuel for the body. Our body only works well if we give it quality fuel.

"RED LIGHT" FOODS TO AVOID

- Sugar

- Red Dye

- MSG

- Processed Foods: Avoid these as much as possible. This necessitates making lunch when possible. Most of the food in school lunches is not nutritious.

- Muffins and Cookies

- Potato Chips

- Fast Food

- Chicken Nuggets: Don't get me started!

- Soda

- Fruit Juice: Yes, even 100 percent pure!

- Candy

- Pizza: Maybe on rare occasions.

- Jelly and Jam

- Hot Dogs: This is pseudo food!

- Cereal

- Dairy

- Peanuts and Peanut Butter: For more details see the NERD NOTE below!

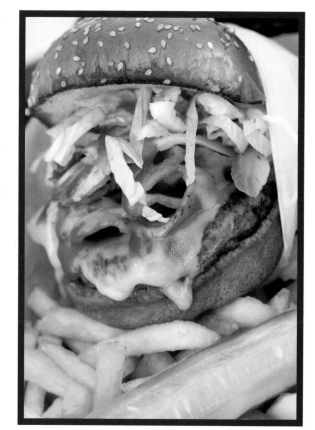

"YELLOW LIGHT" FOODS TO USE IN MODERATION

- Bread: Eliminate white bread as much as possible. Go for whole-grain or Ezekiel bread. I know it's tough, just do your best. Check the nutrition labels for sugar and high fructose corn syrup on the breads that you do buy!

- Pasta: It's basically sugar so try to use Shirataki noodles instead. These are found in the refrigerated section of health food stores. At the very least, use quinoa pasta or whole-wheat pasta. This takes a little longer to digest.

- Oatmeal: This isn't terrible for breakfast, provided that you use steel-cut oats. Rolled or instant oats convert to sugar quickly. Try putting a half scoop of protein powder (I like vanilla-flavored pea protein), chopped nuts or seeds, and some berries in the oatmeal for a more balanced meal. It will give your child focus and energy for a much longer period of time.

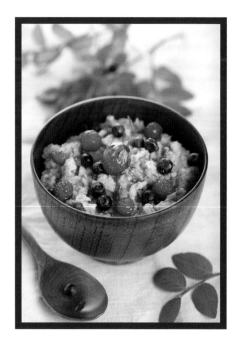

- Freeze-Dried Fruit Snacks with No Sugar Added: These are not Fruit Roll Ups! And they should not be confused with the dried fruit that contains sulfur dioxide. These are a lot lighter. I save these for play dates so I'm not known as the "weird mom" who only serves avocados!

- Baked Sweet Potato Chips: Again, save these for play dates.

- Rice: Use brown rice. White rice is pure sugar. Get them started early on brown rice so they don't notice the difference.

- Corn: For more details see the NERD NOTE below!

Remember, it's always better for your children to eat starchy carbs with some kind of protein so they don't get a bolus of sugar followed by a sharp drop in blood sugar. This affects their focus . . . and their behavior!

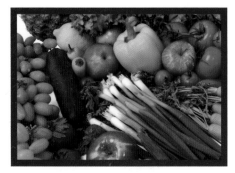

"GREEN LIGHT" FOODS TO CHOW DOWN!

- Veggies, Veggies, Veggies!

- Fruit

- Nuts and Seeds, except peanuts: These are only for children over two years old and for children who don't have allergies.

- Baked Sweet Potatoes

- Brain Boosting Smoothies: These are my favorite treats. They taste great and you can include all kinds of healthy ingredients without your children knowing.

- Raw "Flax Snax": These are great snacks found in the "Raw Food" section of the health food store. These come in many flavors such as pizza, coconut, and chocolate. They are fabulous and nutritious!

- Raw Nut Butters, except peanut butter: These are only for children over two years old and for children who don't have allergies.

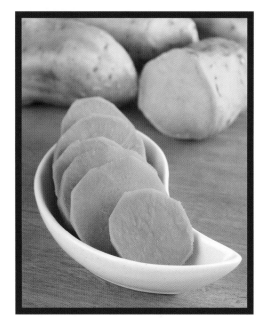

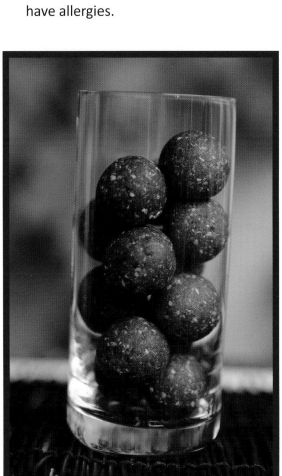

- Wild Fish

- Meat that is lean, grass fed, antibiotic free and hormone free

- Homemade "raw desserts" like "Avocado Gelato" (See page 197 in *Eat healthy With the Brain Doctor's Wife Cookbook.*)

- Raw Macaroons: These are found in the "Raw Food" section of the health food store. You also can make them yourself. (See page 192 in *Eat healthy With the Brain Doctor's Wife Cookbook.*)

Get familiar with your health food store. Most stores have a "Raw Food" section that has great snacks. But beware; some of these snacks are just another marketing scheme for sugary desserts. You have to read the labels!

The Food Trap — Too Bad, So Sad

Peanuts are not nuts. They are actually legumes that are highly susceptible to contamination during growth, storage, and processing (it is very difficult to ensure the proper cleaning of conveyor belts). This leads to infection by the mold fungus, Aspergillus flavus, which releases the toxin . . . **one of the most potent carcinogens.** Peanuts are also very high in omega-6 fatty acids.

Similarly, corn is very high in aflotoxin and in omega-6 fatty acids. Yet, because it is so inexpensive to grow and because it is government subsidized, corn products are in nearly all processed foods in some form or another. This is why you should avoid processed foods as much as possible.

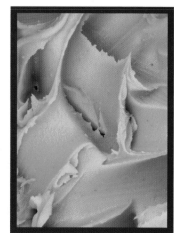

So why, then, are peanuts on the "Red Light" list and corn is on the "Yellow Light" list for what children should eat? This is because it is much easier to eliminate peanut butter and replace it with almond butter or walnut butter whereas corn doesn't have a comparable replacement. Corn is such a common food, liked by most children and found in so many products, that my best suggestion is to limit its consumption. Read ingredient labels and avoid corn oil and additives as much as possible. Corn is best eaten in its "whole" form.

Hopefully, the "Red Light, Yellow Light, Green Light" list makes your life a little easier. You must be committed to giving your children a healthy life, but you must not stress! It's not good for you and it's not good for your kids. Healthy eating has to be a lifestyle, not a chore. In fact, there is much that you can do to alleviate any stress that may occur as you bring your children along on your quest for a life of health and well-being.

As always, you can begin by educating yourself about children and nutrition. When you do, you will see that there even is a biological reason that you may end up locked in a battle of the wills when you ask your child to eat greens! Have you noticed that your kids don't hate all vegetables? Usually it's the really green, bitter ones like spinach, kale, and sometimes broccoli (unless we camouflage the taste). My daughter loves red bell peppers, carrots, squash, cauliflower, and even broccoli . . . pretty much any vegetable except the dark green, leafy ones. This bothered me until I understood the reason. The same qualities in bitter vegetables that make them "good for you" also slow down rapid cell growth. Of course, this is the opposite of what children are doing . . . they are rapidly growing!

It seems that the taste bud receptors for bitter foods usually are not activated until around the time that people stop growing. In general, this is also the time that cancer usually becomes more of a threat . . . and cancer is rapidly growing cells! Apparently, God had a plan!

So, there is no need to get into that battle of wills with your children over vegetables. It is still important for your children to eat vegetables, though, so do your best by being creative, flavoring foods to "taste good," providing less bitter vegetables, and offering fruit. Relax. It will happen when it happens!

Entice Your Children to Love Veggies

- Add greens and other nutritious treats to fruit smoothies. They will never even know!

- Combine greens with another vegetable that your children like.

- Make cauliflower mashed potatoes.

- Make "creamed spinach" with almond milk.

- Add small amounts of veggies to some of their favorite foods.

- Cook veggies more in order to soften them up.

- Be creative with spices, etc.

- Add a little "Earth Balance" to enhance the flavor.

- Use raw almond butter on celery sticks and on red bell peppers.

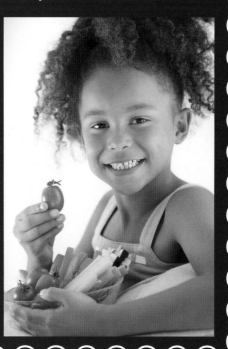

Educating yourself about optimal supplementation for children will also help decrease the stress level over nutrition and whether your kids are getting the "perfect" diet. The reality is, none of us really eat a perfect diet. Basic supplements for children are really important to overall health and brain development.

Daily Supplements for Kids

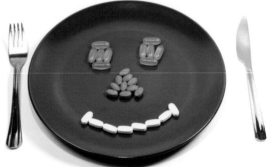

- Multi-vitamin with calcium

- Fish Oil: 1g/day, balanced with EPA and DHA. Some children's formulas have higher levels of DHA for the younger children, but school-age children should get equal amounts.

- Vitamin D: About 1,000 IU/day. While the USRDA is 400 IU, these recommendations are usually quite low. Since vitamin D is a fat-soluble vitamin, be sure to have your child's levels checked if you are ever having his/her blood drawn. Low levels of vitamin D are associated with obesity, depression, and certain types of cancer.

Also, remember that the multi-vitamin you give your child probably has some vitamin D included. Take this into account! Also take into account the amount of time your children spend in the sun and whether or not they wear sunscreen on a consistent basis.

Chloe's Food Game

We play games at the dinner table with our daughter to make learning about nutrition fun. Our favorite is "This Is Good for My Brain, This Is Bad for My Brain." Chloe gives us a "thumbs up" or "thumbs down" sign when we name different foods.

- **Avocados - two thumbs up (God's butter!)**

- **Blueberries - two thumbs up (God's candy!)**

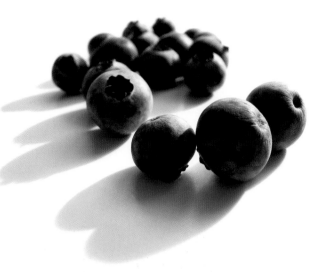

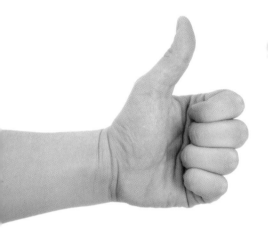

- **Whole-Grain Bread - one thumb up, one thumb down . . . she already knows that bread isn't great, but that whole-grain bread is better than white bread. She often does without the bread.**

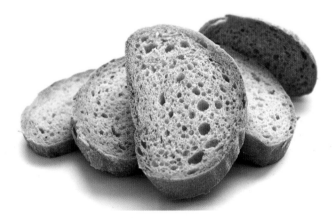

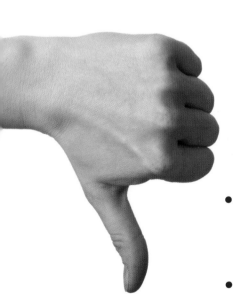

- **Fresh-Squeezed Orange Juice - one thumb down (the sugar). We make a smoothie instead and use the whole orange.**

- **Ice Cream - two thumbs down**

- **Soda - two thumbs down**

The possibilities are endless. Just enjoy yourselves. You never know, you may learn something together!

When all else fails, though, one of the most empowering tools that you have at your disposal is the simple act of allowing your children to make their own mistakes . . . and experience their own consequences. Like many parents, I have found this process to be painful and challenging at times. But, thanks to a great program called "Love and Logic" . . . and the help of my loving husband, I have come to understand that entitled children (or people for that matter) can never be happy. Instead, the best gift that you can give your child is one of empowerment. Unfortunately, the best way to empower a child is to allow them to fall once in awhile. They may experience some pain, but they'll learn the lesson. And though you cannot rescue them, you can be there to hug them. As a wise teacher once said, "Let them learn while the lessons are cheap."

In terms of food and nutrition, they won't always make the choices you want them to make when they are not with you. You can teach them, but they won't always do what you want. Likewise, if you force them, they will likely rebel. But, if you are consistent and get your children invested in their own health as early as possible, you can end up happily surprised by the outcome.

I once read a story about Rhodes Scholars. Apparently, they shared two things in common when they were children. Their parents read to them every night they ate dinner together with their families . . . at the table (not in front of the television). The time we spend with our children is the best investment we can make in their future. How we influence their health while they are young is the greatest long-term gift we can give them. Get them involved in learning about brain health . . . what it means to their life,

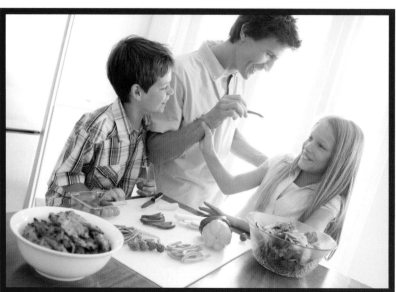 how it helps them, and why it's important. But, above all, teach them that we should give thanks for the food that we are blessed to have and for the nourishment and the energy that this food provides.

Kid Tip:

Have your kids earn their television and/or computer time minute-for-minute by doing physical activity. Better yet, do it with them!

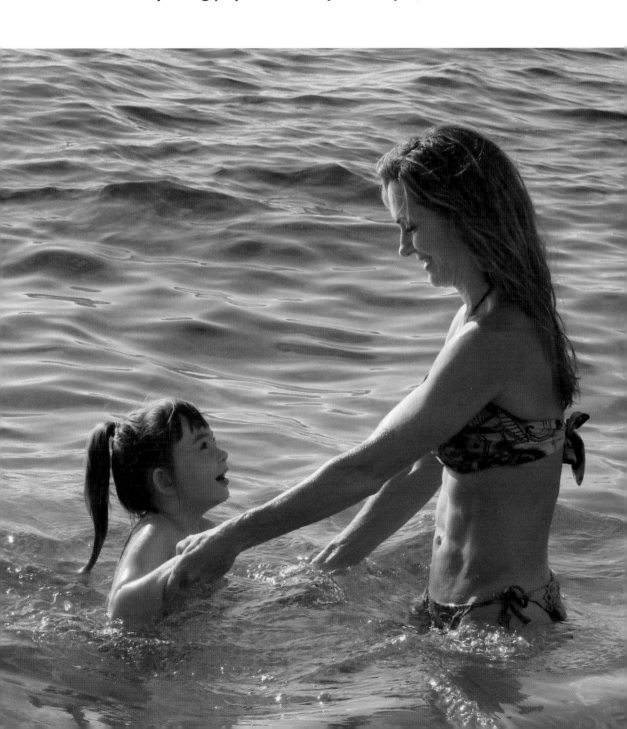

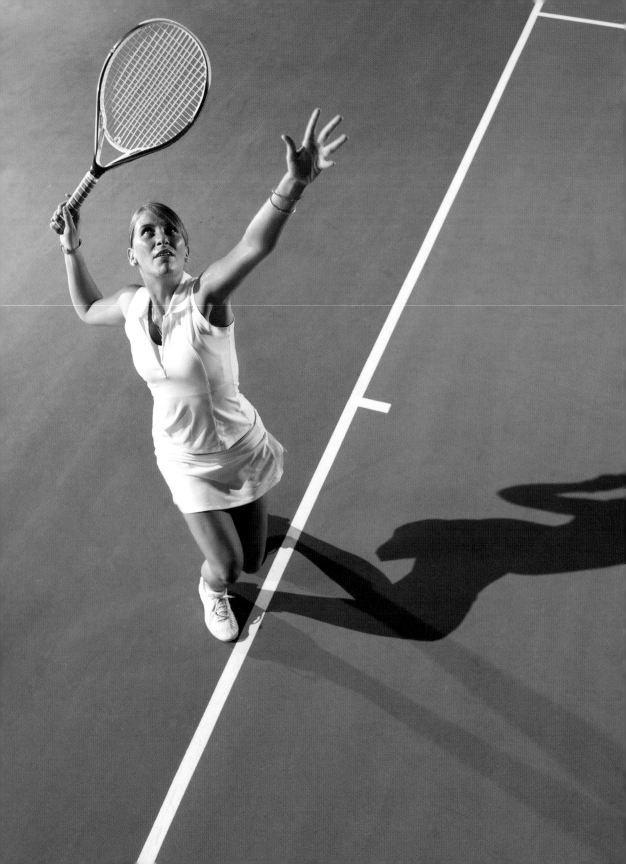

Chapter 11
LET'S GET PHYSICAL: "The Why" and "The How" of Exercise

Chapter 11

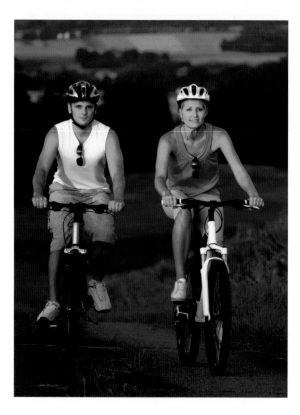

Of the many questions I am asked about fitness, the most common one probably is, "Which is more important when it comes to weight loss, diet or exercise?" The answer is yes! . . . I know, I know. This isn't an answer . . . but that's the point! It is like asking a parent to pick their favorite child. All right, that might be a bad example for some of you, but you get the idea! Even if you have an undisclosed favorite, you know the importance of keeping your family intact and healthy in order for the entire family unit to function normally. Most of you would not say that you love one child better, but you do know that they are different. They each add character and quality to your life in different ways.

But, if you insist on an answer of some kind, I would say that nutrition is technically about 80 percent of the battle of the bulge. However, the 20 percent that is accounted for by exercise is weighted. The amount of good that you do with that 20 percent is monumental.

The reason exercise is important is not because it burns calories! I repeat... You no longer need to read the monitor to see how many calories you burned on the treadmill! If that were the case, many of you would be running your tails off for hours doing penance for just one misstep in your daily routine! It's true that exercise increases metabolism... at least that is the simple answer, and maybe that's all you really need to know. But let's look a little deeper at the importance of exercise:

Exercise: It Does a Body—and a Mind—Good!

- Short-circuits the fat-making cycle (see the "Nerd Note" below).

- Increases insulin sensitivity.

- Decreases systemic inflammation, which reduces joint inflammation and digestive complications.

- Decreases stress and cortisol, one of the leading enemies in the battle of the bulge.

- Increases muscle mass, which requires up to 10 times more energy to function than fat.

- Elevates endorphins in the brain, which is the ultimate "feel-good drug."

- Increases oxygen and other neurophysiological reactions.

- High-intensity, anaerobic, interval training exercise quickly revs the metabolism and burns fat . . . for up to 17 hours after a workout.

NERD NOTE!
"De Novo Lipogenesis" (New Fat Making)

De Novo Lipogenesis refers to the "new fat-making" process that occurs in the TCA cycle, or citrate cycle. We are going to limit our discussion to what happens with sugar, and exercise, to avoid getting too complicated.

I know you're tired of hearing about the evils of fructose, but stick with me just a little longer! We have already established that fructose is fairly toxic for your body. By now you can probably repeat, "Fructose is toxic to the liver" in your sleep. Good! Additionally, when fructose enters the liver there is no release of insulin as there is with glucose. Insulin is what helps us utilize glucose for energy. Without insulin, fructose needs a different vehicle to be converted to usable energy. Something called the "TCA" cycle is initiated to convert the fructose into usable energy in the form of ATP. The end result is carbon dioxide and ATP (we will just refer to ATP as your cellular currency for now). Since fructose is so toxic, its metabolism is very inefficient and there is A LOT of waste product left over in the form of "citrate." This citrate is converted (with the help of three enzymes) to something nasty called VLDL (and a lot of it) or "very low density lipoprotein." VLDL is the bad fat that is responsible for heart disease, making you fat, and bad cholesterol. This is how dyslipidemia (the abnormal amount of fat) is created through fructose consumption. Exercise speeds up the "citrate cycle" and burns off part of the three enzymes before they have the ability to run their normal cycle, thus short-circuiting the fat-making process.

Unfortunately, "de novo lipogenesis" isn't the only nasty thing about fructose consumption. During the TCA cycle there are several other enzymes and phosphates required to contribute the necessary phosphates to fructose. The end result is a waste product called uric acid, which leads to gout and hypertension if enough of it is produced and/or if it is not eliminated effectively.

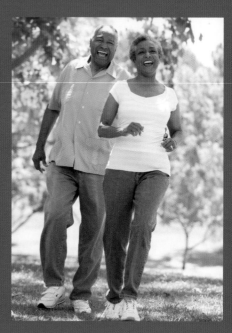

So, there is no doubt that exercise is a key component in a successful fight with the battle of the bulge!

I hope that you now have a clear idea as to why regular exercise is so important. But none of this knowledge will do you any good unless you fully integrate exercise into your lifestyle. You must turn your knowledge into action! That said, I know that getting started on a new exercise routine can seem overwhelming, especially if you have been inactive. And I am going to be presumptuous for a moment and guess that most of you reading this right now are either just getting started in this area of your life or you have not been focusing on your physical health for quite some time. If this is the case, then motivation may be what's holding you back. We all have a million other things that we need to do . . . right?

Wrong! When it comes to exercise, you just have to do it. Fortunately for me, I always have been very motivated to exercise. I have been working out since I was 17 years old, younger if you count high school dance and cheerleading, and I love it. However, it hasn't always been easy to carve out the time for exercise. I have had thyroid cancer, multiple medical issues, a baby, and I was a single, working mother. I was a nurse in a level A trauma unit and I almost never worked regular hours because of nightshifts and overtime. So I know that exercise rarely fits into our lives. But I also know that I have to exercise, so I can be very creative at times.

And if you are creative — and motivated — I bet you can make this happen in your life also! Hopefully, you can find your motivation somewhere within these words, or better yet, within your heart. But, if you do need more motivation, look around you. People who exercise look great and feel great . . . and you knew that before you read this book! But I'm not talking about the airbrushed models who don't eat! That isn't healthy either! I'm talking about health, not advertising. Ask people who you admire for their fitness how they do it. Why do they spend the time they do? How do they find the time? I bet they have the same number of hours in a week that you have, yet they have decided to make exercise one of their primary priorities. Then, if you need even

Leverage Your Motivation

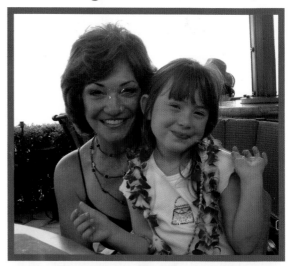

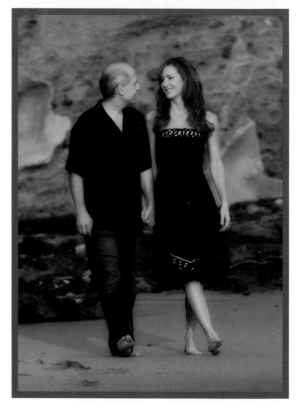

more motivation, look at the people you love. You need to be there to love them, enjoy them, and care for them for as long you possibly can!

A Story About Motivation . . .

One of my favorite stories regarding motivation is about my minister, Rick Warren. I recently was asked to help my husband provide a list of healthy foods to fill the "pastor's lounge" at our church after Rick decided to engage in a lofty project (one of his many) called "Decade of Destiny." Rick's goal with this project is to help his 60,000-member congregation find balance and optimal health in every major area of their lives, including physical health. This is no small task (pun intended)! It requires a monumental commitment from Rick and his staff, not to mention the financial resources he is putting behind his efforts.

To make his vision come to fruition, Rick has gotten my husband, Dr. Daniel Amen, and Doctors Mark Hyman and Mehmet Oz to volunteer their time for this project. The entire congregation will have access to free advice and counseling throughout the year from these three world-renowned doctors. In addition, Rick is building a huge fitness center for the congregation to use free of charge, and he is starting a 170-acre organic farm to supply the restaurants in his five campuses. Leftovers from these restaurants will be donated to the many charities Rick heads up. So what motivates Rick to engage in this massive undertaking? Let me explain . . .

Rick calls his new project "The Daniel Plan." The Bible has a passage (Daniel 1:3-16) in which Daniel has an encounter with Melzar, the chief of staff in charge of training promising new soldiers. These new soldiers are given the "benefit" of being ordered

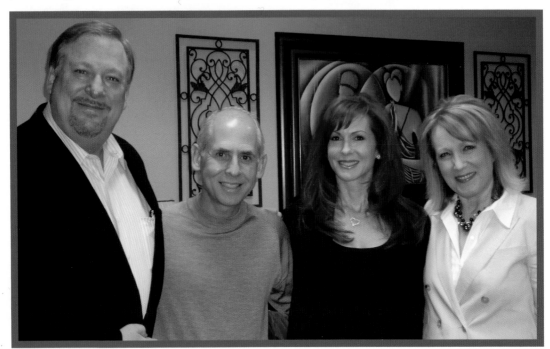

to eat the rich food from the king's table and to drink the king's wine. Daniel was determined not defile his body with the rich foods and wine so he, along with his friends Shadrach, Meshach, and Abednego, asked permission to eat a simple diet of vegetables and water instead. Melzar refused Daniel, so Daniel offered him this challenge:

"Please test us for 10 days on a diet of vegetables and water. At the end of 10 days, see how we look compared to the other young men who are eating from the King's food. Then make your decision in the light of what you see."

The Book of Daniel further explains:

"Melzar agreed to Daniel's challenge and tested them for 10 days. At the end of 10 days, Daniel and his three friends looked healthier and better nourished than the young men who were eating the food assigned by the King. So after that Melzar fed them only vegetables instead of the food and wine provided for the others. God gave these four men an unusual aptitude for understanding every aspect of literature and wisdom."

Rick has struggled with his own weight for years. Yet, his motivation does not come from physical appearance. In his words, "I am already sexy!" His motivation comes from something much deeper. Rick believes that he is commanded by God to take care of the body that God entrusted him with, that his body is the temple of God and that he has been defiling this temple. He also believes that he is the example for his congregation. Once he came to this realization, Rick had no choice other than to get healthy and to help others do the same. It was no longer a "should" . . . It became a "must!"

In Addition to Finding Motivation, You Must Eliminate Excuses.

Here are some ideas:

1. Get your kids to help with housework. (This one is my favorite!)

2. Split the cost of a trainer with a couple of friends. Working out with friends gives you more accountability and makes it more fun.

3. Put a stationary bike or treadmill in front of the television and move your body while you watch your favorite show.

4. Have your kids read to you or do their homework while you work out.

5. Trade child care or meal preparation with a neighbor or friend so you can take turns working out.

6. Join a fun class or hire a trainer to keep you motivated. Many colleges and communities have very inexpensive classes available. Some ideas are yoga, ballroom dancing, tennis, martial arts, swimming, hip hop, etc.

7. Skip cleaning your closet and work out instead. (This one is my second favorite!)

8. Hire an assistant or find a way to trade services with someone to help you for a few hours a week so that you can workout.

9. GET UP AN HOUR EARLIER . . . Of course this means that you may have to go to bed an hour earlier to make sure you get your ZZZ's. In other words . . . I am telling you to prioritize and cut out something else!

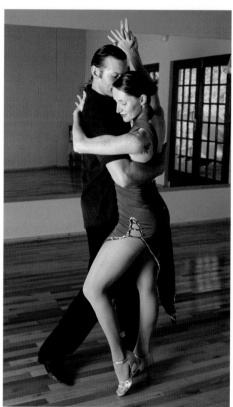

10. Have a stack of interesting books to read while you are on the stationary bike. Have audiobooks already downloaded on your iPod for while you walk. Have your TiVo'd shows or your DVDs ready to watch while you work out. In other words, make your workout time a time that you look forward to!

I came up with these 10 ideas in five minutes! Right now, I want you to write down 10 ideas that work for your lifestyle. This is only your life we are talking about! Find the time to exercise for at least 30 minutes a day now or you will have plenty of time... when you are dead. The first few days may take some effort but, after 30 days, I promise that you never will want to give it up!

What are the best ways to work out?

There is some debate about the best way to exercise. For those of you raised in the legwarmer and leotard age, you think cardio, cardio, cardio when you think of exercise. But, gone are the days of spending hours on the StairMaster or treadmill (YEAH!!!). Research now shows that long-distance running and hours spent doing aerobics actually have many negative affects on the body. Chronically training in an aerobic style decreases muscle mass, increases cortisol, and depletes organ reserves (which are important to have if you are ever ill or injured). This is good news for you!

Current research shows that the most effective and healthiest forms of exercise are shorter in duration yet higher on the intensity scale. Even better, there are many variations of this training so there is a little something for everyone! No matter what, though, if you never have engaged in regular physical exercise or if you have an underlying medical condition you must consult your physician before starting any new program. These variations include:

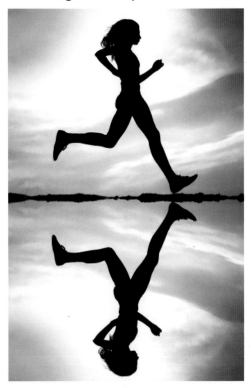

1. Interval Training: This type of exercise is all about working at a moderate pace, then going all out for a "burst" of greater intensity, then returning to the initial pace repeatedly throughout the duration of your training time. For example, you can walk like you are late for a few minutes, sprint for a "burst," walk for a few minutes, sprint for a "burst," and so on. You also can do this while riding a bike, walking on a treadmill, riding an exercise bike, etc. These bursts should last from 30 seconds to 1 minute, and you should not exceed 30 minutes for your total training time.

2. Circuit Training: This type of training routine is all about combining high-intensity aerobic output with resistance exercises. For example, you can exercise with dumbbells for 10 repetitions then immediately move to the next exercise or aerobic activity and so on. You will move from exercise to exercise until you complete a circuit (which generally consists of anywhere from three to 10 exercises depending on your fitness level and goals). Then, after completing a circuit, you generally rest for about 1 minute and repeat the cycle (the actual length of your rest time and the number of circuits that you complete also are determined by your fitness level). I like this style of training for many people. It is efficient and it builds strength and endurance.

3. Alternating Strength Training with Anaerobic Interval Training: This is, by far, my favorite way to exercise. You do need to invest 20-40 minutes a day for 4-6 days each week, but the gains you make far exceed this investment in time. For 2-3 days per week, you perform heavy strength training. For the other 2-3 days per week you do the "Interval Training" described above in order to rev up your metabolism.

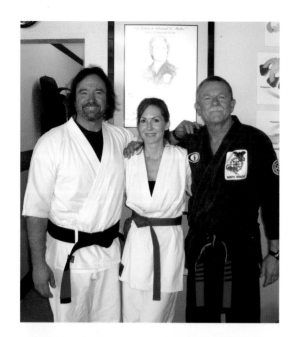

4. Coordination Exercises: These types of exercises help to stimulate the cerebellum, which is the portion of your brain that is responsible for coordination. This includes martial arts (as long as you don't sustain a brain injury), yoga, choreographed dance with complex moves, and any other exercise that requires you to constantly learn and to perform complex movements on both sides of your body.

Muscle Madness

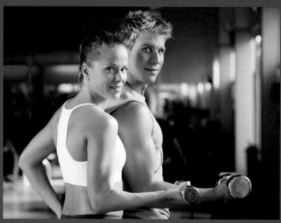

- Muscle is 18 percent more dense than fat, which means that as you lose weight and gain muscle you have the added benefit of looking more "compact."

- Lean muscle mass requires more energy to maintain your body's basic energy needs, or metabolism, . . . up to 10 times more energy than fat. This may not seem like much if you are thinking in terms of 1 pound of muscle (20 extra calories burned) compared to 1 pound of fat (2 or 3 calories burned). But, if you take into consideration the entire body composition, packing on lean muscle mass really adds up. An extra 200 calories burned each day adds up to 1,400 calories each week, 6,000 calories each month . . . or 73,000 calories each year! That's about 20 pounds per year. Just from pumping a little iron!

- Lean muscle mass *will not increase your overall size* when it is compared to fat. Losing fat and increasing lean muscle mass will decrease your size by up to 18 percent per pound of fat. You will be *solid and toned!*

- It's a myth that putting on muscle will make you gain weight and make you bulky (unless you are Arnold training to be Mr. Olympia) . . . especially if you are female. It will take a LONG time and great genetics before you work out enough to take off the weight and add enough muscle to make enough of a difference that you will have to buy bigger clothes! I wish it were that easy... believe me, I try! I challenge you to do it. If I'm wrong, e-mail me. I want to know your secrets.

- If you have fat to lose, more muscle will help you reach your goal more quickly.

- Lean muscle mass is one of the main predictors of longevity. Most people begin a rapid decline in overall muscle mass by the time they are in their 30s or 40s. This decline in muscle mass actually begins a signaling process in your genes. Your body starts to think that you are slowing down and not of much use to the species anymore. I know this sounds harsh, but if you are not able to help the species survive, there isn't much reason to keep you around. Of course I'm being a bit dramatic for effect—and it is more complicated than that when metabolic reserve, organ reserve, inflammatory responses, and hormonal influences are taken into account—but this is the short version.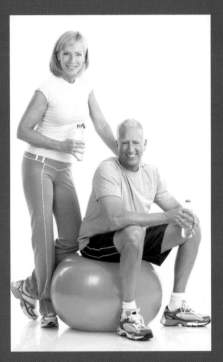

- Strength training and weight lifting, which increase muscle mass, help to maintain bone density and prevent osteoporosis.

- You will look sexy in your jeans. Notice, this is last on the list! Nonetheless, it's true and it's certainly an important motivating factor for many of you!

Putting It All Together

As with all of the healthy eating information that you have learned in this book, **there comes the moment when learning turns into doing.** However, when it comes to exercise, I know that many of you are beginners or you are coming back to exercise after a long hiatus. Below, you will find an introductory workout that I have written for you. For those of you who are more accustomed to exercise (and as beginners progress), the intensity of this routine easily can be adapted to your fitness level. Even better, this workout routine has been created so that you don't need to belong to a fancy gym.

There is a way to exercise with virtually no equipment. I have intentionally modified this routine so that you can work out from

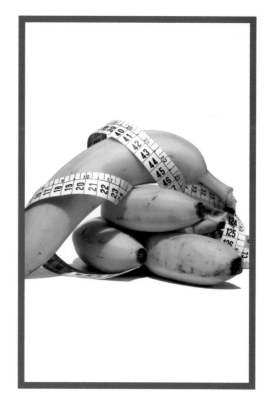

home, on the road or nearly anywhere. If you can afford it, I recommend purchasing a set of dumbbells and a bench. If you don't have the money for a bench, a chair will do. If you don't have the money for the dumbbells, you can make due without them until you find the resources to invest in some.

The thing I most highly recommend for beginners, though, is a heart-rate monitor. If you can't afford one, be sure you monitor your heart rate manually and do it regularly throughout your routine! Once you are in shape, this won't be as critical. But, when you are first starting, you must make sure that you are not going beyond a level that is safe!

Also, when you start exercising, you might find that you feel so good that you get excited and really motivated. Do NOT take this as a sign to go crazy . . . one of the fastest ways to achieve results is to NOT over-train! You don't need to train longer, you need to train smarter!

For my suggested workout, you will do Strength Training on Monday, Wednesday, and Friday for approximately 40 minutes each day. For this, you will use body weight or dumbbells. You will do Interval Training on Tuesday, Thursday, and Saturday for approximately 20-30 minutes each day, but no longer. For this, you will walk like you're late for something important for 3 minutes and you will follow this with a "burst" of maximum exertion for 30 seconds to 1 minute, depending upon your fitness level. This will be different for everyone. Try to "burst" at least four times during your walk.

If you are just starting and overweight, your pace for your Interval Training may be barely fast enough to be considered walking. That's all right. You aren't being graded. If you are in decent shape and just want to lose a few pounds, you may be sprinting uphill. Great! It is what it is, and you are doing something!

The following is an ideal schedule, but if you only work out 4-5 days a week you still will get results. Just remember, your results are in direct correlation to the amount of *effort* that you invest. The schedule looks something like this:

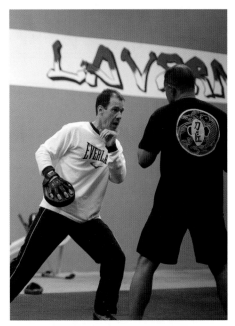

Photo by Chris Worden

The Routine:

Monday: Strength Training. Use the workout template included (see appendix 3 on page 196).

Tuesday: Interval Training for 30 minutes (20 minutes initially). Wear your heart-rate monitor!

Wednesday: Strength Training. Use the workout template (see appendix 3 on page 196).

Thursday: Interval Training for 30 minutes (20 minutes initially). Wear your heart-rate monitor!

Friday: Strength Training. Use the workout template included (see appendix 3 on page 196).

Saturday: Go for a leisurely walk for 30 minutes... or you can do Interval Training if you wish.

Sunday: Rest and Rejuvenate.

Tana's Workout Description

Special thanks to my trainer, Brad Davidson, from Stark Training for his help designing a safe introductory workout that can be done anywhere! For more information on Stark Training and Brad Davidson, please visit www.starktraining.com.

First Things First: Warm-up and Range-of-Motion Criteria

It's essential that you begin any workout routine with a proper warm-up and with a Range-of-Motion (ROM) routine. There are a plethora of warm-up routines that you can practice and most will serve you well. However, my advice to you is to keep your warm-up simple. Begin by walking or by riding an exercise bike at low resistance for 5-10 minutes. This will help to increase your body temperature and your heart rate in a gentle way. Also, this will help get your muscles loose and your body ready for exercise.

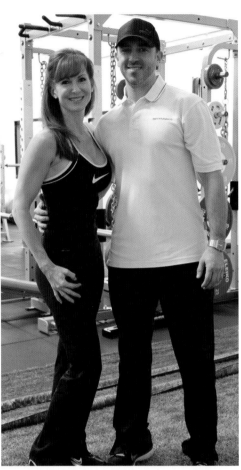

Next, do some Range-of-Motion exercises such as head rotations, shoulder rolls, small arm-circles, gentle side bends and forward bends, hip rotations, knee rotations, hamstring stretches, calf stretches, etc. You get the idea. Always move gradually and comfortably and increase your range of motion without using any ballistic or bouncy movements. All of your movements and stretches should be done in a manner that is smooth and gentle while also warming up your muscles and joints. This will help prepare you for exercise.

Post Workout = Cool Down

After every workout, take 5-10 minutes to do a proper cool down. This easily can be done by taking a slow walk or by riding a stationary bike with very little resistance. This cool down period is essential for bringing your heart rate down to its normal level in a gentle and gradual manner. Don't skip the cool down!

The Workout

Split Squat (Lunges)

[Equipment Needs: None]

You get a lot of bang for your buck with lunges, which target all the big muscles in your legs including the calves, hamstrings, quadriceps, inner and outer thighs, hips and glutes (the behind). That's a lot of muscles to work with one simple move.

Start by standing with your feet hip-width distance apart.

1. Step your left foot back about 2 feet so you are resting on the ball of the left foot. Make sure your front foot is completely flat on the floor.

2. Slowly bend both knees and lower your body into a lunge so your left knee is almost touching the ground and your right knee is in line with or slightly behind your right toes. Keep your torso upright rather than leaning forward.

3. Come back to standing.

4. Do 15-20 reps on each side.

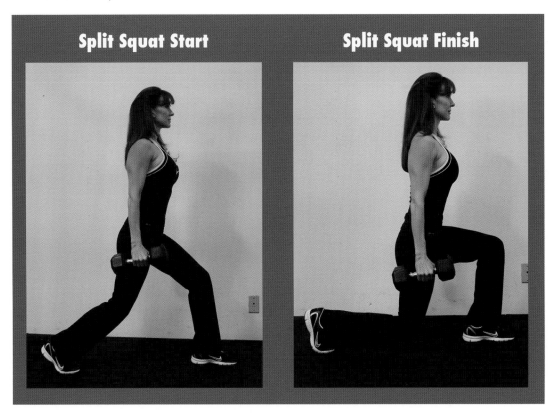

Split Squat Start   Split Squat Finish

Dumbbell Single Arm Rows

[Equipment Needs: Dumbbells (women start with 5-10 pounds, men start with 10-15 pounds) and a bench/couch/bed]

If you've ever leaned over to pick up something off the floor, you've done a single arm row. Rows may look like they're targeting your arm muscles, but they actually are strengthening the muscles in your back.

1. Start with your left knee and left hand on a bench (or you can use a couch or bed) and your back parallel to the floor. Hold a free weight in your right hand, making sure it is in alignment with your right shoulder.

2. Bend your right elbow as you slowly pull the weight toward you, making sure you don't hunch your shoulder up toward your ear.

3. Do 10-12 reps.

4. Switch sides so your right knee and right hand are on the bench/couch/bed and the weight is in your left hand.

5. Do 10-12 reps.

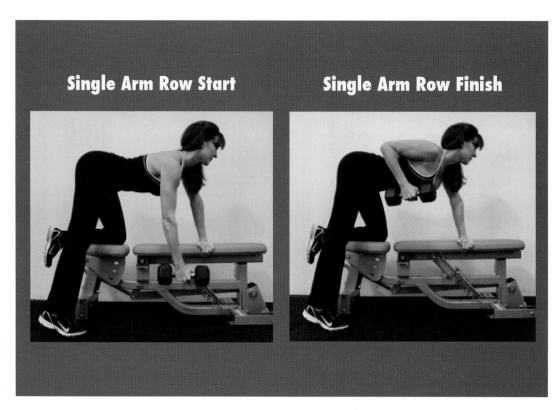

Single Arm Row Start   **Single Arm Row Finish**

Bridge with Alternating Leg Lifts

[Equipment Needs: None]

This is a great lift to really tone and tighten the glutes (the behind) without the risk of hurting your back.

1. Start by lying on your back with both your knees bent and your feet flat on the floor. Allow your arms to rest on the ground at a 45-degree angle (this is for support and to aid in balance).

2. Push through your heels and lift your hips up towards the ceiling.

3. Really squeeze your abs and slowly lift your right foot about 6 inches off the ground. Slowly lower your foot back to the ground. Switch to lifting your left foot about 6 inches off the ground. (To make this exercise more difficult, extend the leg you are lifting straight out.)

4. Perform 15-20 lifts on each leg.

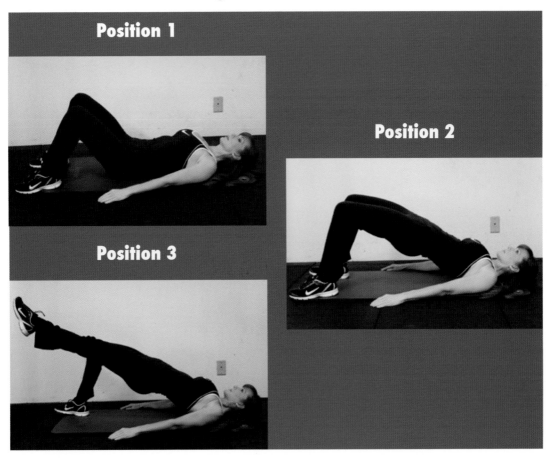

Position 1

Position 2

Position 3

Chest Press

[Equipment Needs: Dumbbells (women start with 5-8 pounds, men start with 12-15 pounds)]

This upper-body move targets the chest muscles.

1. Lie on your back with your feet on the floor and your knees bent.

2. Holding your dumbbells, put your arms out to your sides, and bend your arms at a 90-degree angle to the floor.

3. Lift the weights straight up toward the ceiling, keeping your hands in alignment with your shoulders. Exhale as you lift.

4. Bend your elbows and lower the weights in a slow and controlled motion back down to the starting position.

5. Do 10-12 reps. If you can do more than 12 reps easily, the weight isn't heavy enough. If you can't do 10 reps, switch to lighter weights.

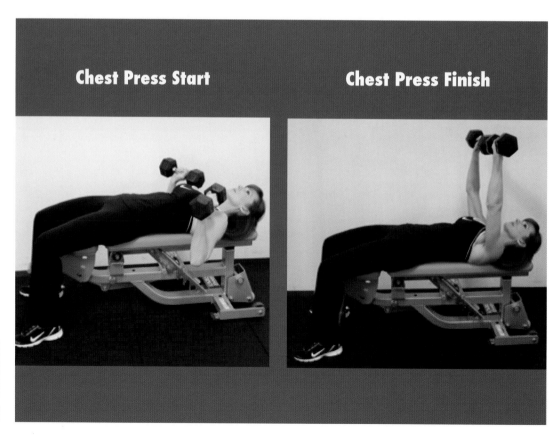

Chest Press Start   Chest Press Finish

Plank Rolls

[Equipment Needs: None]

This move may look like it focuses on your arms, but it also targets your core muscles. This is essential for having a strong abdomen and a healthy back.

1. Lie face down on the ground and rest your forearms on the floor so that your right hand is near your left elbow and your left hand is near your right elbow.

2. Lift your body up so you are supporting your body weight on your forearms and your toes.

3. Pull your abs in and hold your body straight without letting your backside pop up in the air or letting your middle sag down toward the ground. Hold this position for 8 seconds.

4. Keeping your right arm bent, twist your body to the right so your right side is facing the ceiling. Don't let your hips sag down toward the ground. Hold this position for 8 seconds.

5. Twist back down to the start position. Hold this position for 8 seconds.

6. Keeping your left arm bent, twist your body to the left so your left side is facing the ceiling. Don't let your hips sag down toward the ground. Hold this position for 8 seconds.

7. Start with 2-4 reps (1 rep = face down, right and left position). Eventually, work up to 12 reps.

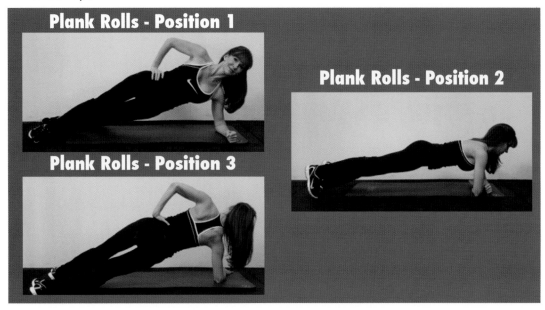

Plank Rolls - Position 1

Plank Rolls - Position 2

Plank Rolls - Position 3

Bird Dog

[Equipment Needs: None]

This is one of the best and safest core exercises to help strengthen the muscles that help to protect the spine.

1. Start on your hands and knees. You want your hands to be in alignment with your shoulders and your knees to be in alignment with your hips. Make sure your eyes are looking straight at the ground and try really hard to keep your head in alignment with your body.

2. Slowly lift your right hand off the ground and extend it out at a 45-degree angle while, at the same time, you lift your left knee off the ground and extend your left leg out straight.

3. Hold both limbs off the ground for 5 seconds then place the hand and the knee back on the ground.

4. Now repeat with your left hand and your right knee.

5. Do 4 reps each side. Eventually, work up to 10-12 reps on each side.

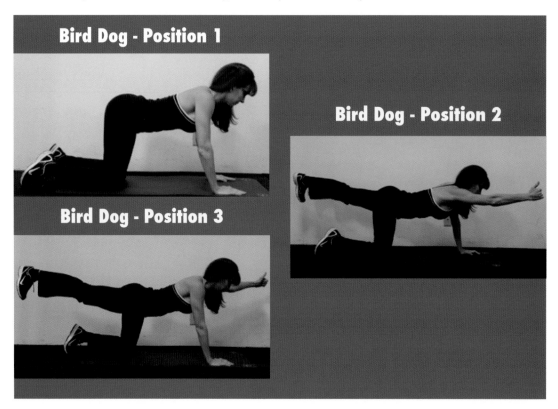

Bird Dog - Position 1

Bird Dog - Position 2

Bird Dog - Position 3

A Note About Training Safely . . .

For all of these exercises, be sure to rest between sets until your heart rate comes back to your target heart range. For strength training this is 60 percent of your maximum heart range. To figure your target heart range:

- Determine your maximum heart range by subtracting your age from 220. For cardio your target heart rate is usually around 70 percent of maximum. For interval training your heart rate may temporarily reach up to 85 percent of your maximum heart rate, but it will not be sustained before you decrease your intensity and recover.

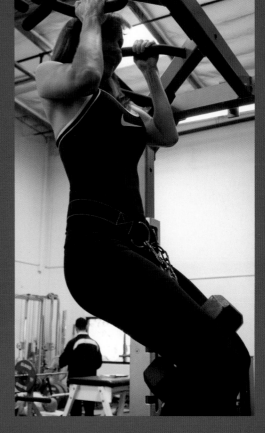

- Multiply your maximum heart range by .60. This is your target heart range. This number can increase a bit as your fitness level increases. It also may be a little lower if you have specific health issues (check with your physician).

Also, as you begin to increase your strength and endurance, you will naturally decrease the amount of rest time between sets. You then may begin to add exercises that engage multiple major muscle groups such as push-ups and pull-ups. When you really get into shape, you also may wish to incorporate "bursting" segments into your strength workout. I do a workout similar to this when I travel, but I do calisthenics, squat-thrusts or running on stairs between sets. Always be sure to rest until your heart rate comes back to your target heart range before starting a new set.

Train safely . . . and enjoy your new energy and vitality!

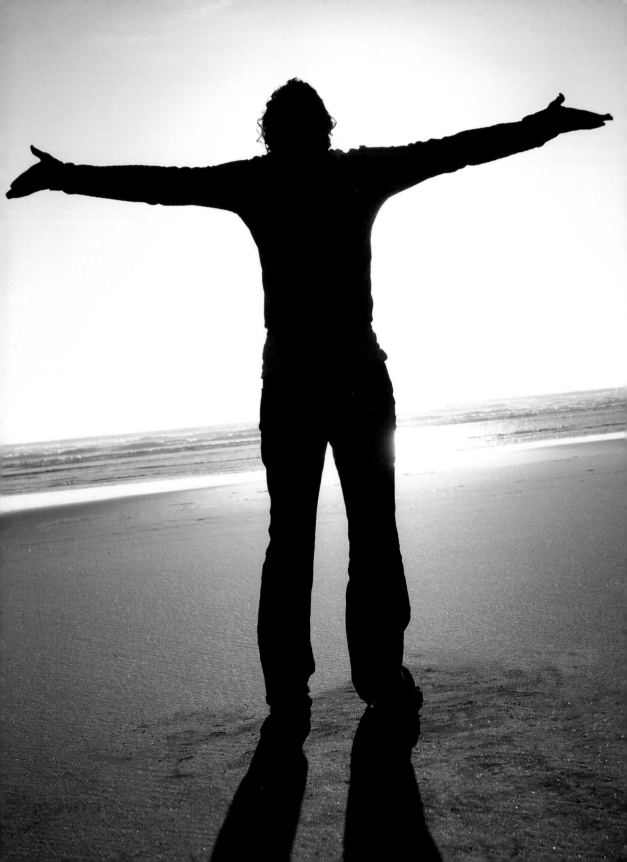

Chapter 12

SAMPLE MENU: Two Weeks to Jump-Start Your New Life

TWO-WEEK SUCCESS MENU

Chapter 12

This two-week sample menu will help get you started on your journey to success. The recipes are found in the *Eat healthy With the Brain Doctor's Wife Cookbook*. This menu is to help you see just how often you should be eating and just how diverse your menu really can be! This is not deprivation! This is not boring! This is healthy, energizing eating! With a little creativity, there are as many options as there are days in a year.

But, if you are anything like me, you probably are pretty busy and on the run! In all honesty, I don't eat this way every day. My menu is a bit less complex than what I am offering you here. I am a creature of habit and my staple foods don't change much . . . LOTS OF VEGETABLES! But, the meal that is always diverse in our house is dinner. Plus, when we make dinner, we make sure to make enough food so that I automatically have lunch made for the next day. That saves me a lot of time.

I have been called the "food police" more than once, so I want to be careful to meet you where you are and not go overboard. Many of these recipes are versatile so you can adapt them according to where you are on your journey. If you aren't quite ready to ditch all bread and refined carbs, you may eat some of the wraps and burgers with buns or tortillas. But, as you progress, try eating them "open faced" (half the bread) or with lettuce wraps instead. It is really important that you take this step because cutting as much bread and refined carbs out of your diet as early in your program as possible is the surest way to jump-start your weight loss. Remember, these refined carbs are literally the drug that controls your hormonal balance. And, within a week of not eating them, you likely will not miss them at all!

*The portion sizes are adjustable according to individual dietary and metabolic needs and activity level. If you need to "beef" up your calorie count a bit, add another half portion to one or two of the meal items. Men may need to double the portion sizes on some meal items.

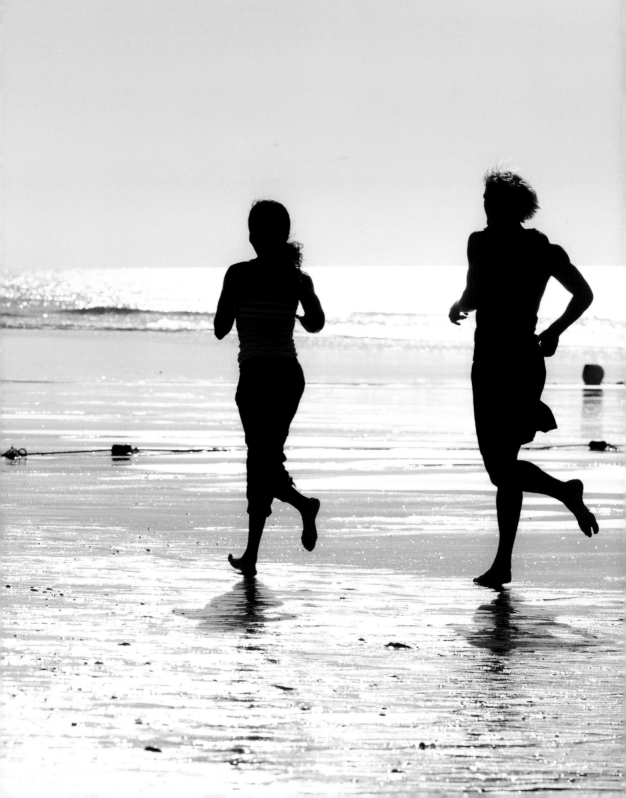

Tana's Menu Tips

Tip 1: Eat breakfast within one hour of waking.

Tip 2: Meals should be about three hours apart. You should not let yourself get hungry.

Tip 3: Measure all portions according to the recipes in the cookbook section.

Tip 4: Women should eat protein portions approximately 3-4 oz in size, or 15-20 grams.

Tip 5: Men should eat protein portions approximately 4-6 oz in size, 20-25 grams.

Tip 6: If there is not a nutritional chart available, estimate portion sizes by using the palm of your hand. Your protein portion should not exceed the size of the palm of your hand, including depth.

Tip 7: Try to limit breads and refined carbohydrates as much as possible for the first two weeks in order to break your addiction to sugar.

Tip 8: Make your carbs "whole" or "sprouted grains" as much as possible. This includes quinoa, brown rice, barley, farro, steel cut oats, etc.

Tip 9: Eat grains like a condiment. Limit all grain consumption to no more than ½ cup servings at one time. Your body can process this amount easier.

Tip 10: Eat some protein and healthy fat with grains to slow down absorption of sugar.

Tip 11: Try eating sandwiches "open faced" (with one piece of bread only).

Tip 12: Never use white bread.

Tip 13: Try to use Ezekial bread when possible. It is sprouted grain and flourless.

Tip 14: If using hamburger buns, use Oroweat Multi-Grain Sandwich Thins® brand. It is thin and only has 100 calories for both sides (less than half the calories). Even better if you eat it open faced.

Tip 15: Drink 16 oz of water before meals.

Tip 16: Eat the salads listed below with 1 tablespoon of oil and either some balsamic vinegar or some lemon juice.

Tip 17: The nuts and seeds are strategically placed in the menu plan to help increase satiety, boost omega 3 fatty acids, and prevent gluconeogenesis (the conversion of muscle to glucose during weight loss).

Tip 18: If you still feel hungry, increase your raw vegetable intake. They are nearly "free" calories. It takes almost as much energy to digest them as they contain. And you get the benefit of a gazillion micronutrients. It's NOT the same with fruit!

Tip 19: If you really, REALLY are going to cheat, do it with protein. Don't do it with carbs. I repeat... DO NOT cheat with carbs even though they may count for equal or less calories. Calories are not equal in this game. Protein will increase satiety and drive insulin down. Carbs will cause insulin to rise.

Tip 20: By necessity, the vegetarian meals contain more grains and carbs. We have used as little as we could get away with, though. It's a balancing act between this and not using too much soy. My suggestion to vegetarians is to eat a whole lot of raw and lightly cooked vegetables, to use only a little in the way of grains and tofu, and to increase things like nuts, hemp, chia seeds, etc. There may not be quite as much variety in your meal plan, but what you eat will be nutritious, delicious, and vitalizing. Make Shirataki noodles one of your staples! You can dress them up with a thousand combinations.

Tip 21: Most of the recipes give options to use Shirataki noodles instead of pasta. I strongly suggest this! This is free calories (it is virtually calorie free), compared to pasta, which is loaded with calories and carbs (aka sugar). These will fill your tummy without bankrupting your calorie allowance.

Tip 22: When possible, use a couple Romaine lettuce leaves for "wraps" instead of tortillas or pitas.

Tip 23: Don't view the reduction in carbs as deprivation. Your calorie intake isn't changing just because we removed the carbs. If you cut out the bread you get to add more protein, nuts or even a little fruit. These things will do far more to nourish you and increase your feeling of satisfaction.

WEEK 1 SUCCESS MENU

	BREAKFAST	SNACK	LUNCH
DAY 1	Berry Alert Brain-Boosting Smoothie	¼ cup raw almonds or sunflower seeds	Amazing Apple Cinnamon Chicken Salad
DAY 2	Feel-Good Eggs Ranchero	½ cup berries	Seared Ahi with Cucumber Salad
DAY 3	Green Apple Goddess Brain-Boosting Smoothie	¼ cup raw nuts or seeds	Mixed green salad with grilled chicken breast with 1 tablespoon olive oil and balsamic
DAY 4	Guilt-Free Granola	Low-carb protein bar	Get Fit Fennel and Orange Salad with added chicken breast
DAY 5	Very Omega Cherry Brain-Boosting Smoothie	¼ cup nuts or seeds	Spinach and Strawberry Salad with Pecans with added shrimp
DAY 6	Coco Chunky Monkey Brain-Boosting Smoothie	Chopped veggies with Surprising Split Pea Hummus	Tasty Turkey Wrap
DAY 7	Seafood Omelet for Super Focus with ¼ cup berries	¼ cup raw nuts or seeds	Stay Sharp Chard Salad with added chicken breast

WEEK 1 SUCCESS MENU

SNACK	DINNER	DESSERT
2 cups mixed veggies with 2 tablespoons hummus	The Best Beef Stroganoff	2 oz. Amazing Avocado Gelato
Large mixed green salad with 1 tablespoon seeds and 1 tablespoon olive oil & lemon juice	Sizzling Chicken and Veggie Kabobs	¼ cup Fruit Granita
1 crisp pear and 2 tablespoons raw nuts or seeds	"Spaghetti" with Turkey Meatballs and steamed broccoli	Brain on Joy bar available at www.amenclinics.com
½ cup berries of your choice and ¼ cup raw almonds	Simple Shrimp Scampi and Vegetable Soup	½ oz. extra dark chocolate (NOT MILK CHOCOLATE)
2 cups raw vegetables with 2 tablespoons guacamole	Memory-Boosting Eggplant Moussaka with 2 cups steamed vegetables	Grilled Peaches (no more than one peach)
1 apple and ¼ cup raw nuts or seeds	Crowd-Pleasing Cioppino	Blueberry Cobbler (1 serving)
1 sliced tomato with avocado (about 2 tablespoons)	Chicken Marsala with Roasted Brussels Sprouts & Large green salad with 1 tablespoon balsamic vinaigrette	Magnificent Chocolate Macaroons (1 each)

WEEK 2 SUCCESS MENU

		BREAKFAST	SNACK	LUNCH
DAY 1		Totally Tofu Scramble	1 apple and 1 low-carb protein bar	Get Smart Mahi Mahi Burger (with low-carb, whole-grain bun or wrapped in Romain lettuce)
DAY 2		Tropical Storm Brain-Boosting Smoothie	2 cups chopped veggies with 2 tablespoons baba ghanouj	Avocado Wrap with added turkey
DAY 3		Brainy Breakfast Burrito (consider wrapping in Romaine lettuce)	1 apple and ¼ cup raw nuts or seeds	Rainbow Quinoa Salad with added chicken breast
DAY 4		Sunrise Surprise Brain-Boosting Smoothie	2 cups raw veggies with ¼ cup guacamole	Peaceful Asian Pear Salad with added shrimp
DAY 5		Alpha Omega Oatmeal	Large green salad with tomatoes, 1 tablespoon olive oil and lemon juice and 1 tablespoon sunflower seeds	Low-Cal Lo Mein with Veggies with added shrimp
DAY 6		Chocolate-Covered Strawberry Brain-Boosting Smoothie	1 sliced tomato with sliced avocado (about 2 tablespoons)	Lemon Pepper Halibut with 1 head steamed broccoli
DAY 7		Gluten-Free Pancakes with Blueberries and Banana (1 small one) with 1 egg	2 cups veggies with 2 tablespoons hummus or Surprising Split Pea Hummus	Chicken Vegetable Wrap

WEEK 2 SUCCESS MENU

SNACK	DINNER	DESSERT
Green salad with 1 tablespoon olive oil and lemon juice	Pan Roasted Salmon with Vegetables	2 oz. Amazing Avocado Gelato
¼ cup raw nuts and seeds and ½ cup seeded grapes	Savory Lubian Rose Stew (brown rice optional, not suggested)	Warm Sweet Potato Pudding
Low-carb protein bar	Brain Fit Fajita Salad	½ cup Chocolate Mousse
Low-carb protein bar	Teriyaki Rice Bowl with Salmon	½ oz. extra dark chocolate (NOT MILK CHOCOLATE)
1 pear with ¼ cup raw nuts or seeds	Baked Salmon with Roasted Leeks	Grilled Peaches (1 each)
1 apple with ¼ cup raw nuts or seeds	Indian-Style Chicken with Creamy Broccoli Soup and green salad with 1 tablespoon vinaigrette dressing	Brain on Joy bar available at www.amenclinics.com
½ cup berries with ¼ cup raw nuts	Shirataki Noodles with Edamame and Smoked Salmon	Magnificent Chocolate Macaroons (1 each)

WEEK 1 SUCCESS MENU: VEGETARIAN

	BREAKFAST	SNACK	LUNCH
DAY 1	Berry Alert Brain-Boosting Smoothie	¼ cup raw almonds or sunflower seeds	White Bean Soup for the Wise
DAY 2	Feel-Good Eggs Ranchero	½ cup berries	Arugula Salad with Raspberries and Hemp Seeds with added tofu
DAY 3	Green Apple Goddess Brain-Boosting Smoothie	¼ cup raw nuts or seeds	Very Veggie Pita
DAY 4	Guilt-Free Granola	Low-carb protein bar	Get Fit Fennel and Orange Salad with added tofu
DAY 5	Very Omega Cherry Brain-Boosting Smoothie	¼ cup nuts or seeds	Spinach and Strawberry Salad with Pecans with added tempeh
DAY 6	Coco Chunky Monkey Brain-Boosting Smoothie	Chopped veggies with Surprising Split Pea Hummus	Rainbow Quinoa Salad with seeds
DAY 7	Seafood Omelet for Super Focus with ¼ cup berries	¼ cup raw nuts or seeds	Stay Sharp Chard Salad with added tempeh

WEEK 1 SUCCESS MENU: VEGETARIAN

SNACK	DINNER	DESSERT
2 cups mixed veggies with 2 tablespoons hummus	Energizing Chipotle Enchiladas (2)	2 oz. Amazing Avocado Gelato
Low-carb protein bar	Veggie Kabobs, Mung Bean Salad with 2 tablespoons mixed flax, hemp, and chia seeds	1/4 cup Fruit Granita
1 crisp pear and 2 tablespoons raw nuts or seeds	"Spaghetti" and steamed broccoli	Brain on Joy bar available at www.amenclinics.com
½ cup berries of your choice and ¼ cup raw almonds	Tempeh with Vegetables	½ oz. extra dark chocolate (NOT MILK CHOCOLATE)
2 cups raw vegetables with 2 tablespoons guacamole	Barley Veggie Bowl with Sweet Potatoes with extra steamed veggies	Grilled Peaches (no more than one peach)
1 apple and ¼ cup raw nuts or seeds	Grilled Polenta with Roasted Beans	Blueberry Cobbler (1 serving)
1 sliced tomato with avocado (about 2 tablespoons)	Sinless Spinach Lasagna with Roasted Brussels Sprouts and a large green salad with 1 tablespoon balsamic vinaigrette	Magnificent Chocolate Macaroons (1 each)

WEEK 2 SUCCESS MENU: VEGETARIAN

	BREAKFAST	SNACK	LUNCH
DAY 1	Totally Tofu Scramble	1 apple and 1 low-carb protein bar	Portobello Burger (with low-carb, whole-grain bun)
DAY 2	Tropical Storm Brain-Boosting Smoothie	2 cups chopped veggies with 2 tablespoons baba ghanouj	Avocado Wrap with added tofu and seeds if desired, but there should be enough protein as is
DAY 3	Brainy Breakfast Burrito (consider wrapping in Romaine lettuce)	1 apple and ¼ cup raw nuts or seeds	Rainbow Quinoa Salad with added tempeh
DAY 4	Sunrise Surprise Brain-Boosting Smoothie	2 cups raw veggies with ¼ cup guacamole	Grilled tofu and green salad with 1 tablespoon olive oil and lemon juice
DAY 5	Alpha Omega Oatmeal	2 cups veggies with 2 tablespoons hummus or Surprising Split Pea Hummus	Low-Cal Lo Mein with Veggies
DAY 6	Chocolate-Covered Strawberry Brain-Boosting Smoothie	1 sliced tomato with sliced avocado (about 2 tablespoons)	Keen Quinoa Pilaf with steamed broccoli
DAY 7	Gluten-Free Pancakes with Blueberries and Banana (1 small one) with 1 egg	Large green salad with tomatoes, 1 tablespoon olive oil and lemon juice and 1 tablespoon sunflower seeds	Lentil Pilaf

WEEK 2 SUCCESS MENU: VEGETARIAN

SNACK	DINNER	DESSERT
Green salad with 1 tablespoon olive oil and lemon juice	You'll Never Know It's Vegetarian Chili	2 oz. Amazing Avocado Gelato
¼ cup raw nuts and seeds and ½ cup seeded grapes	Vegetarian Savory Lubian Rose Stew	Peach Coconut Cream Dream
Low-carb protein bar	Brain Fit Fajita Salad with tempeh instead of chicken	½ cup Chocolate Mousse
Low-carb protein bar	Teriyaki Rice Bowl with tempeh instead of salmon	½ oz. extra dark chocolate (NOT MILK CHOCOLATE)
1 pear with ¼ cup raw nuts or seeds	Pasta Pomodoro and Easy Eggplant Parmesan with sautéed wax beans and baby bok choy	Grilled Peaches (1 each)
1 apple with ¼ cup raw nuts or seeds	Sinless Spinach Lasagna with Creamy Broccoli Soup and green salad	Brain on Joy bar available at www.amenclinics.com
1 cup berries with ¼ cup raw nuts	Shirataki Noodles with Edamame and tofu	Magnificent Chocolate Macaroons (1 each)

APPENDIX 1: GLYCEMIC INDEX (GI)

Low GI: 55 and under   Medium GI: 56 to 69   High GI: 70 and above

Glycemic Index Ratings

Grains	Glycemic Index
French baguette	83 ± 6
White bread	75 ± 2
Whole wheat bread	74 ± 2
White rice	72 ± 8
Bagel, white	69
Brown rice	66 ± 5
Couscous	65 ± 4
Hamburger bun	61
Basmati rice	57 ± 4
Quinoa	53
Spaghetti, white	49 ± 3
Pumpernickel bread	41
Barley, pearled	25 ± 2

Breakfast Foods	Glycemic Index
Scones	92 ± 8
Instant oatmeal	79 ± 3
Cornflakes	77
Waffles	76
Froot Loops	69 ± 9
Pancakes	66 ± 9
Kashi Seven Whole Grain Puffs	65 ± 10
Bran muffin	60
Blueberry muffin	59
Steel-cut oatmeal	52 ± 4
Kellogg's All-Bran	38

Fruit	Glycemic Index
(raw unless otherwise noted)	
Dates, dried	103 ± 21
Watermelon	80 ± 3
Pineapple	66 ± 7
Cantaloupe	65
Raisins	64 ± 11
Kiwi	58 ± 7
Mango	51 ± 5
Banana, overripe	48
Grapes	43
Nectarines	43 ± 6
Banana, underripe	42
Oranges	45 ± 4
Blueberries	40
Strawberries	40 ± 7
Plums	39
Pears	38 ± 2
Apples	36 ± 5
Apricots	34 ± 3
Peach	28
Grapefruit	25
Cherries	22

Vegetables	Glycemic Index
Instant mashed potato	87 ± 3
Baked potato	86 ± 6
Sweet potato	70 ± 6
French fries	64 ± 6

Sweet corn	52 ± 5	Milk, full fat	41 ± 2
Peas	51 ± 6	Skim milk	32
Carrots, boiled	39 ± 4	Tomato juice	31
Yam	35 ± 5		
Artichoke	15	**Snack products**	**Glycemic Index**
Asparagus	15		
Broccoli	15	Tofu-based frozen dessert	115 ± 14
Cauliflower	15		
Celery	15	Pretzels	83 ± 9
Cucumber	15	Puffed rice cakes	82 ± 10
Eggplant	15	Jelly beans	80 ± 8
Green beans	15	Licorice	78 ± 11
Lettuce	15	Pirate's Booty	70 ± 5
Peppers	15	Angel food cake	67
Snow peas	15	Popcorn	65 ± 5
Spinach	15	Water crackers	63 ± 9
Squash	15	Ice cream	62 ± 9
Tomatoes	15	Potato chips	56 ± 3
Zucchini	15	Snickers bar	51
		Milk chocolate, Dove	45 ± 8
Legumes and Nuts Index	**Glycemic**	Corn chips	42 ± 4
		Low-fat yogurt	33 ± 3
Baked beans, canned	40 ± 3	M&Ms peanut	33 ± 3
Chickpeas	36 ± 5	Dark chocolate, Dove	23 ± 3
Pinto beans	33	Greek-style yogurt	12 ± 4
Butter beans	32 ± 3	Hummus	6 ± 4
Lentils	29 ± 3		
Cashews	25 ± 1	**Meals**	**Glycemic**
Mixed nuts	24 ± 10	**Index**	
Kidney beans	22 ± 3	McDonalds hamburger	66 ± 8
		Pizza Hut vegetarian supreme, thin, and crispy	49 ± 6
Beverages Index	**Glycemic**		
Gatorade, orange flavor	89 ± 12		
Rice milk	79 ± 8		
Coca-Cola	63		
Cranberry juice	59		
Orange juice	50 ± 2		
Soy milk	44 ± 5		
Apple juice, unsweetened	41		

Sources: This list of foods and their GI is culled from numerous sources, including a 2008 review of nearly 2,500 individual food items by researchers at the Institute of Obesity, Nutrition and Exercise in Sydney, Australia.

Get screening laboratory tests and your blood pressure tested to optimize your brain and body. Here are tests normally ordered at the Amen Clinics for our weight loss groups. Ask your health care provider to order these as part of a healthy brain/body program.

- **Complete Blood Count**—to check the health of your blood. People with low blood count can feel anxious and tired, and may overeat as a way to medicate themselves. People with alcohol problems may have large red blood cells.

- **General metabolic panel**—to check the health of your liver, kidneys, fasting blood sugar, and cholesterol. Normal total cholesterol is less than 200.

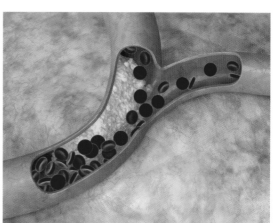

LDL (the bad cholesterol)-

Normal is 70- 130 mg/ dl

HDL (the good chlolesterol)-

Normal is 46- 199 mg/ dl

Triglycerides-

Normal is 0- 150 mg/ dl, Optimal is less than 100

*An important ratio is the Triglyceride (TG)/ HDL ratio. If you divide your level of TG by the HDL, it should be under 4 (ideally). If it is above 4, it is a sign that you are developing toxicity and inflammation!

- **Cortisol** is a stress hormone whose primary function is to increase blood sugar, suppress immune function, and aid in the metabolism of proteins, fats, and carbohydrates. Elevated levels of cortisol may be an indication of poor sleep, excessive stress, insulin resistance, trauma, too much caffeine, problems with immunity, or certain diseases associated with the adrenal glands.

Normal Cortisol levels range between 4.0- 22.0 mcg/ dl

- **Fasting Insulin** is an early indicator of inflammation. It is also used to detect insulin resistance. Chronically elevated levels of insulin have been associated with obesity, metabolic syndrome, various types of cancer, PCOS, hypertension, and heart disease.

  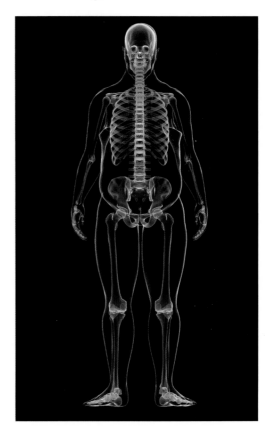

  Ideal Fasting Insulin is below 5 uU/ ml.

  The upper limit of "normal" is 10 uU/ ml.

- **AA/EPA ratio** is an early indicator of inflammation. It tells you the ratio of fatty acids in your system.

  Normal is 3.0. Ideal is 1.5.

  Above 3.0 is a sign of inflammation.

  Above 12 may be a sign of toxicity.

At the Amen Clinics, most of the people we see have a ratio over 20. The overweight and chronically ill people often have ratios as high as 40!

- **Vitamin D level**—Have your physician check your 25-hydroxy vitamin D level, and if it is low get more sunshine and/or take a vitamin D3 supplement. I have to take 10,000 international units of Vitamin D3 a day to keep my levels near high normal.

  Low < 30

  Optimal 50-90

  High > 100

- **Thyroid**—An overactive thyroid can mimic symptoms of anxiety that make you want to eat as a way to calm down. Having low thyroid levels decreases overall brain activity, which can impair your thinking, judgment, and self-control, and make it very hard for you to lose weight. Have your doctor check your free T3 and TSH levels to check for hypothyroidism or hyperthyroidism and treat as necessary to normalize.

- **C-reactive protein**—This is a measure of inflammation that your doctor can check with a simple blood test. Elevated inflammation is associated with a number of diseases and conditions and should prompt you to eliminate bad brain habits and get thin. Fat cells produce chemicals called cytokines that increase inflammation in your body.

  Normal is <0.1

- **HgA1C**—This test shows your average blood sugar levels over the past two to three months and is used to diagnose diabetes and prediabetes.

  Normal results for a nondiabetic person are in the range of 4 to 6 percent.

  Prediabetes is indicated by levels in the 5.7 to 6.4 percent range.

  Numbers higher than that may indicate diabetes.

- **DHEA and free and total serum testosterone level**—Low levels of the hormones DHEA and testosterone, for men or women, have been associated with low energy, cardiovascular disease, obesity, low libido, depression, and Alzheimer's disease.

- **Blood pressure**—Have your doctor check your blood pressure at your yearly physical or more often if it is high. High blood pressure is associated with lower overall brain function, which means more bad decisions.

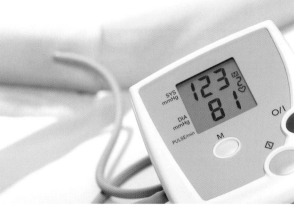

  Normal blood pressure is considered 120/80, but can be variable according to fitness level and individual health considerations.

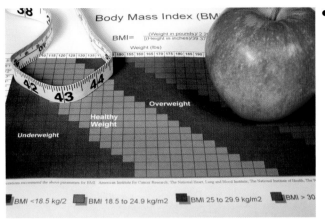

- **Body Mass Index (BMI)**— This number tells you the health of your weight compared to your height.

  Normal: between 18.5 and 25

  Overweight: between 25 and 30

Obese: between 30 and 40 is obese

Morbidly Obese: over 40

To be healthy, happy, and smart, you have to get your BMI under control. For a free BMI calculator go to www.amenclinic.com.

- **Waist to Height Ratio (WHtR)** – Another way to measure the health of your weight is called your waist to height ratio. Some researchers believe this number is even more accurate than your BMI. BMI does not take into account an individual's frame, gender, or the amount of muscle mass versus fat mass. For example, two people can have the same BMI, even if one is much more muscular and carrying far less abdominal fat than the other; this is because BMI does not account for differences in fat distribution.

  The WHtR is calculated by dividing waist size by height, and takes gender into account. As an example, a male with a 32 inch waist who is 5'10" (70 inches) would divide 32 by 70, to get a WHtR of 45.7 percent. The WHtR is thought to give a more accurate assessment of health since the most dangerous place to carry weight is in the abdomen. Fat in the abdomen, which is associated with a larger waist, is metabolically active and produces various hormones that can cause harmful effects, such as diabetes, elevated blood pressure, and altered lipid (blood fat) levels.

  Many athletes, both male and female, who often have a higher percentage of muscle and a lower percentage of body fat, have relatively high BMIs but their WHtRs are within a healthy range. This also holds true for women who have a "pear" rather than an "apple" shape.

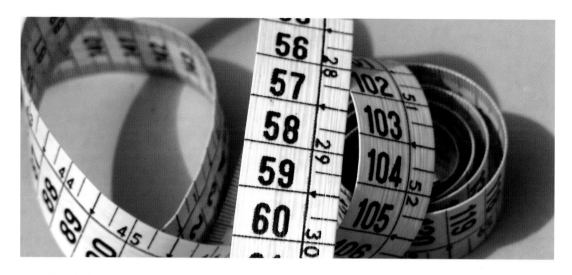

The following chart helps you determine if your WHtR falls in a healthy range (these ratios are percentages):

Women:

Ratio less than 35: Abnormally Slim to Underweight

Ratio 35 to 42: Extremely Slim

Ratio 42 to 49: Healthy

Ratio 49 to 54: Overweight

Ratio 54 to 58: Seriously Overweight

Ratio over 58: Highly Obese

Men:

Ratio less than 35: Abnormally Slim to Underweight

Ratio 35 to 43: Extremely slim

Ratio 43 to 53: Healthy

Ratio 53 to 58: Overweight

Ratio 58 to 63: Extremely Overweight/Obese

Ratio over 63: Highly Obese

- **Know how many of the twelve most important modifiable health risk factors you have**, then work to decrease them. Here is a list from researchers at the Harvard School of Public Health. Circle the ones that apply to you.

  Smoking

  High blood pressure

  BMI indicating overweight or obese

  Physical inactivity

  High fasting blood glucose

  High LDL cholesterol

  Alcohol abuse

  Low omega-3 fatty acids

  High dietary saturated fat intake

  Low polyunsaturated fat intake

  High dietary salt

  Low intake of fruits and vegetables

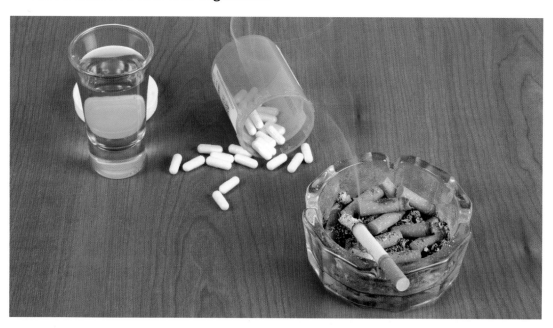

Using the moves described on pages 167 - 173, I have created the following workout routine for you.

Here's how to read the following workouts. These workouts involve "supersets," which means you do A1, rest for the recommended number of seconds, then do A2, rest, then go back to A1. You do all sets of A1 and A2 then move onto the B exercises then the C exercises.

For example, your Week 1 workout would go as follows.

A1. Split Squat	15-20 reps	rest 120 seconds
A2. DB Single Arm Row	10-12 reps	rest 120 seconds
A1. Split Squat	15-20 reps	rest 120 seconds
A2. DB Single Arm Row	10-12 reps	rest 120 seconds
B1. Bridge with Alternating Leg Lifts	15-20 reps	rest 120 seconds
B2. Chest Press	10-12 reps	rest 120 seconds
B1. Bridge with Alternating Leg Lifts	15-20 reps	rest 120 seconds
B2. Chest Press	10-12 reps	rest 120 seconds
C1. Plank Rolls	1 each	rest 100 seconds
C2. Bird Dog	2 each	rest 100 seconds
C1. Plank Rolls	1 each	rest 100 seconds
C2. Bird Dog	2 each	rest 100 seconds

Workout:

A1 Split Squat

Week	Sets	Reps	Rest (seconds)
1	2	15-20	120
2	2	15-20	100
3	3	15-20	90
4	3	15-20	75

A2 DB Single Arm Row

Week	Sets	Reps	Rest (seconds)
1	2	10-12	120
2	2	10-12	100
3	3	10-12	90
4	3	10-12	75

B1 Bridge with Alternating Leg Lifts

Week	Sets	Reps	Rest (seconds)
1	2	15-20	120
2	2	15-20	100
3	3	15-20	90
4	3	15-20	75

B2 Chest Press

Week	Sets	Reps	Rest (seconds)
1	2	10-12	120
2	2	10-12	100
3	3	10-12	90
4	3	10-12	75

C1 Plank Rolls

Week	Sets	Reps	Rest (seconds)
1	1	1 each (hold 8 secs)	100
2	2	2 each (hold 8 secs)	90
3	3	2 each (hold 8 secs)	75
4	3	3 each (hold 8 secs)	60

C2 Bird Dog

Week	Sets	Reps	Rest (seconds)
1	1	2 each (hold 5 secs)	100
2	3	3 each (hold 5 secs)	90
3	3	3 each (hold 5 secs)	75
4	3	4 each (hold 5 secs)	60

Change Your Brain Change Your Body by Daniel G. Amen, M.D.

Dr. Gundry's Diet Evolution by Steven R. Gundry, M.D., F.A.C.S., F.A.C.C.

Toxic Fat by Barry Sears, PH.D

The Paleo Diet by Loren Cordain, Ph.D.

The Paleo Solution, The Original Human Diet by Robb Wolf

Ultra-Metabolism by Mark Hyman, M.D.

Nutrition for the Focused Brain and the Recovering Brain by Jeffrey L. Fortuna, DR. P.H., M.S.

The End of Overeating by David A. Kessler, M.D.

Genetic Roulette by Jeffrey M. Smith

You on a Diet by Michael F. Roizen, M.D., and Mehmet C. Oz, M.D.

Healing ADD by Daniel G. Amen, M.D.

Personal Power (audio) by Anthony Robbins

"Doctors Warn Avoid Genetically Modified Food" by Jeffrey M. Smith (Online at http://www.articles.mercola.com, March 25, 2010)

"Drug Company Owns Monsanto and Their Weed Killer Is What Funds GMO Crops" by David Barboza, *The New York Times*

"Sugar: The Bitter Truth" by Robert Lustig, M.D., USSF Professor Of Pediatric

Division Of Endocrinology, UC Television

Perfect Girls, Starving Daughters by Courtney E. Martin

Dying To Be Thin by Ira M. Sacker, M.D., and Marc A. Zimmer, Ph.D.

Regaining Your Self by Ira M. Sacker, M.D., and Sheila Buff

The Eating Disorder Sourcebook, Third Edition by Carolyn Costin, M.A., M.Ed., M.F.T.

The Courage To Heal, Third Edition by Ellen Bass and Laura Davis

Loving What Is by Byron Katie with Stephen Mitchell

Parenting With Love and Logic by Foster Cline, M.D., and Jim Fay

ACKNOWLEDGMENTS

It is with gratitude and love that I first would like to thank my husband, Daniel. Your tremendous support, encouragement, and faith in me give me the energy and the drive to deliver this message of health and healing. You are my best friend and partner!

Special thanks go to Jaclyn Frattali for her amazing work on the book design and graphics. Jim Kennedy, a wonderful photographer and artist, you were a pleasure to work with and a true professional.

To Brad Davidson, my personal trainer, I would like to offer thanks and recognition. Brad trains many high-level athletes, yet he was never too busy to help design safe protocols for our clients and friends. You are one of the most knowledgeable trainers I know when it comes to special needs related to injury and when it comes to advanced training protocols.

I'd like to give special thanks to Kamila Reschke, our chef and friend, for helping to keep our family healthy. Kamila was my partner in writing the cookbook companion to this book.

Special recognition and thanks go to Melissa Ryan for her tremendous help and support with the editing process. Your writing skills and perseverance were an invaluable asset to the timely completion of this project. Thank you for your outstanding effort and achievement.

George Ryan, a trusted friend was also a tremendous help in consulting and research. George is an officer for the Los Angeles Police Department's "Special Weapons And Tactics" unit. He is also a trainer for CrossFit, an outstanding martial artist and long-time fitness enthusiast. Thank you for your time and attention to detail, and for your training advice.

I'd also like to thank Frances Sharpe for her tremendous contribution to research and editing. Frances is a wonderful writer and always a pleasure to work with.

Thanks to my beautiful daughter Chloe for being an unending source of joy and inspiration. I love you with my whole heart!

I am grateful to my best friend, Jeana, and to my sisters for their undying support and for allowing me to continually read them my new material.

Of course, I am eternally grateful to my mother for the life she gave me. I only hope to look half as vital and youthful as she does when I'm in my sixties!

ABOUT THE AUTHOR

Tana K. Amen graduated magna cum laude from Loma Linda University with a Bachelor of Science Degree in Nursing and has worked as a Trauma/Neurosurgical ICU nurse.

Tana is a health enthusiast and has been focused on fitness for over two decades. She also worked with some of the sickest patients in the hospital and saw the effects of poor lifestyle choices and the intense need for special nutrition when patients were healing from brain injuries and other traumas.

In spite of her medical and fitness background, Tana was repeatedly surprised when her own health failed her throughout the years. She was diagnosed with thyroid cancer at the age of 23. How could someone who lived a consciously healthy lifestyle be diagnosed with cancer and the numerous other health issues that presented themselves over the years? That's when she began to further her education about nutrition and the role it plays on overall health.

Tana began to realize that "health" and "fitness" are not synonymous. Furthermore, she came to the conclusion that many of the basic nutrition principles she had learned in her youth were outdated and not enough to optimize wellness in a person's life. There is a major difference between sustenance and optimal nutrition for a high-energy, passionately healthy lifestyle!

Tana is the nutrition and fitness leader of the Amen household. She practices martial arts regularly, has a black belt in Tae Kwon Do, and enjoys a variety of other physical activities, including tennis and weight lifting. Keeping her family focused on fitness and health is a primary value for Tana.

ABOUT AMEN CLINICS, INC.

Amen Clinics, Inc. (ACI) specializes in helping people heal from behavioral, learning, emotional, cognitive, and weight issues for children, teenagers, and adults. ACI has an international reputation for evaluating and treating:

- **Attention Deficit Disorder (ADD)**
- **Anxiety**
- **Depression**
- **School Failure**
- **Brain Trauma**
- **Obsessive Compulsive Disorders**
- **Bipolar Disorder**
- **Aggressiveness**
- **Marital Problems**
- **Substance Abuse**
- **Obesity**
- **Alzheimers Disease and Memory Loss**

Brain SPECT imaging is one of the tools used by the Clinics. ACI has the world's largest database of brain SPECT scans related to behavioral problems. ACI welcomes referrals from physicians, psychologists, social workers, marriage and family therapists, drug and alcohol counselors, and individual clients.

Clinic Locations:

Southern California
4019 Westerly Place, Suite 100
Newport Beach, CA 92660

Pacific Northwest
616 120th Ave NE, Suite C100
Bellevue, WA 98005

Northern California
1000 Marina Blvd, Suite 100
Brisbane, CA 94005

East Coast
1875 Campus Commons Drive #101
Reston, VA 20191

Visit www.amenclinics.com or call 888-564-2700 for a consultation.

Amenclinics.com is an educational, interactive brain website geared toward mental health and medical professionals, educators, students, and the general public. It contains a wealth of information to help you learn about our clinics and the brain. The site contains over 300 color brain SPECT images, thousands of scientific abstracts on brain SPECT imaging for psychiatry, a brain puzzle, and much, much more.

Visit Dr. Amen's new online solution that will hold your hand and give you all the tools you need to get thinner, smarter, and happier NOW, including:

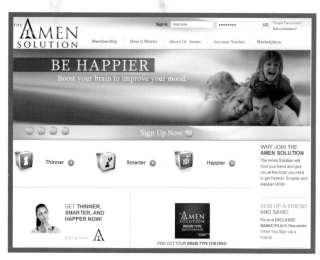

- Detailed questionnaires, to help you know your BRAIN TYPE and personalize this program to your own individual needs. You will also be able to test your memory and get a personalized plan to get thinner, smarter, happier, AND learn how to decrease your risk of Alzheimer's disease.

- There is an interactive daily online journal to track your important numbers, calories, and brain healthy habits, like sleep and exercise – THIS IS THE SINGLE MOST IMPORTANT TOOL FOR IMPROVING YOUR HEALTH.

- There are hundreds of brain healthy recipes, tips, shopping lists, and menu plans.

- Plus, you will get an exclusive, award winning 24/7 BRAIN GYM MEMBERSHIP where you can test, work out, and strengthen your brain to reduce stress, improve your memory and attention, and boost your mood. It is like having a personal trainer for YOUR OWN BRAIN. You will learn how your own brain works, train it specifically to fit your needs, and optimize your life. The brain gym has been described as "wildly fun...the positive thinking exercises have carried me through the day...."

- In addition, we will send you daily tips and even text messages to help you remember your supplements and stay on track to get healthy NOW.

- And whenever you feel sad, mad, nervous, or out of sorts, we will have exercises to help you boost your mood, decrease depression and help you feel better fast.

- Plus much, much more.

- The online program is your personal guide to getting thinner, smarter, and happier.

ABOUT AMEN CLINICS